Pure Substances and Mixtures

Author
Ted Gibb

Program Consultant
Marietta (Mars) Bloch

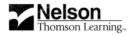

Nelson
Thomson Learning™

Australia • Canada • Denmark • Japan • Mexico • New Zealand • Philippines
Puerto Rico • Singapore • South Africa • Spain • United Kingdom • United States

Pure Substances and Mixtures

Contents

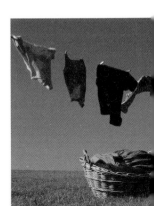

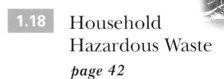
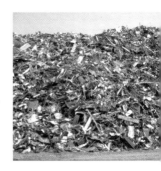
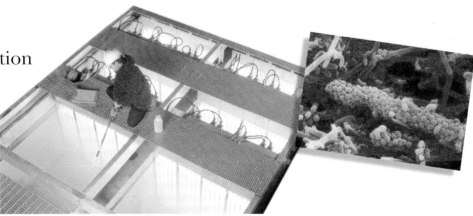

Important safety information

Record observations or data

Refer to numbered section in
Nelson Science & Technology 7/8
Skills Handbook

Unit 1 Overview

atter is all around us: the air we breathe, the lakes and oceans, and Earth itself are all made of matter. To manufacture things or make them useful to us, we work with matter in all sorts of ways: we purify matter to obtain metals, mix up other types of matter to make foods or drinks, and we separate manufactured items to recycle the parts. But how do we know which substances will mix well for a particular purpose? Can we classify matter in a way that will help us make predictions?

Classifying Matter

Matter can be classified into many different categories. This helps us make sense of the thousands of different substances around us.

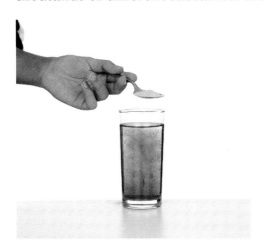

You will be able to:

- distinguish between pure substances and mixtures

- investigate different methods of separating the components of mixtures

- use the particle theory to explain how substances dissolve

- conduct experiments to determine the factors that affect the rate at which substances dissolve

- describe the difference between saturated and unsaturated solutions

Using Matter to Make Products

The products that we use in our everyday lives make use of the physical properties of the substances they are made from.

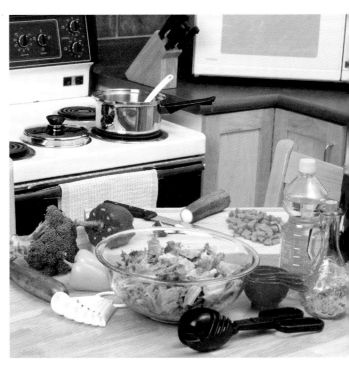

You will be able to:

- distinguish between raw materials and processed materials

- describe how raw materials are collected and processed to produce products

- identify a variety of manufactured products made from mixtures and explain their functions

- recognize that solutions in manufactured products can exist as solids, liquids, and gases

Sustainability Concerns

The use of large amounts of raw materials from the Earth to manufacture a wide range of products has an impact on the environment, the economy, and our health. Our environment is affected by manufacturing and agricultural processes. It needs to be protected by regulations and public awareness programs.

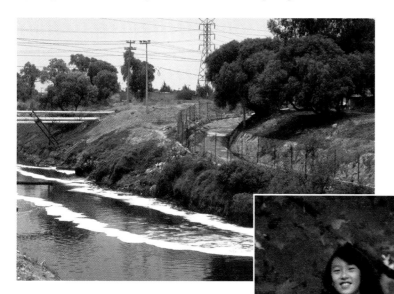

You will be able to:

- identify the sources and characteristics of pollutants that result from manufacturing and chemical fertilizers

- describe the effect of some toxic solvents on the environment, and regulations that ensure their safe use and disposal

- identify different types of waste present in the community and methods of disposal

- evaluate the quality of water from different sources by performing simple tests

Design Challenge

You will be able to ...
demonstrate your learning by completing a Design Challenge.

A System That Separates or Purifies Materials

Recycling substances and products, both liquid and solid, is an important way of preserving Earth's resources and reducing garbage. However, recycling and separating substances also requires many types of technology.

In this unit you will be able to design and build:

1 A Water Purification System
Design and build a model of a filtering system that removes solid particles from water.

2 A Recycling System for Plastic, Glass, Metal, and Paper
Design and build a model in which plastic, glass, metal, and paper items are separated from each other.

3 A Soil and Gravel Mechanical Separator
Design and build a model that efficiently separates soil and rocks into three different sizes.

To start your Design Challenge, see page 54.

Record your thoughts and design ideas for the Challenge when you see

Design Challenge

Getting Started

What Are Things Made Of?

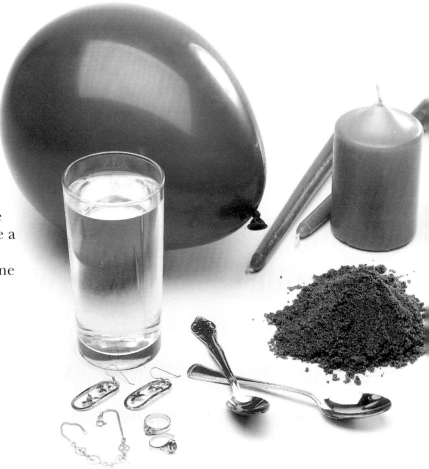

1 We can see and feel most types of matter. We can also describe them in many different ways — for example, soft, hard, shiny, colourful, brittle, liquid, solid. Some things, like air, we cannot see or taste. Why is it important to have a way to classify things? Which classification system is best? Does one classification work for everything?

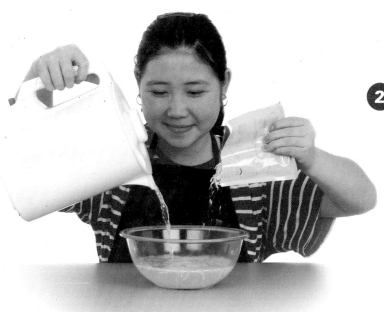

2 To make products, we mix raw materials together in combinations that may require heating, freezing, stirring, melting, hardening, or dissolving. Through a series of processes, we end up with the items that we buy and use every day. How do we know which materials mix best to give us the product we want? How do we decide which is the best process to use when manufacturing a product?

3 The raw materials we use to make products all come from the Earth. Some, like our food, we grow. Others, like metals and other minerals, we mine. And when we don't want something anymore, or it breaks, we throw it away. Both retrieving substances from the Earth and throwing things into landfills have an effect on the environment. How can we lessen this effect and create a balance between environmental concerns, health concerns, and economic concerns?

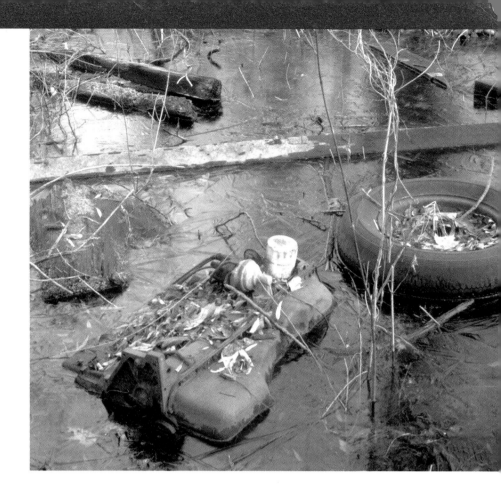

Reflecting

Think about the questions in **1**,**2**,**3**. What other questions do you have about mixtures? As you progress through this unit, reflect on your answers and revise them based on what you have learned.

Try This Classifying Candy

Examine some chocolate candy bars and organize them into categories.

• Using a dinner knife, cut each candy bar into pieces.

1. Does each candy bar look the same throughout, or can you see other substances mixed in?

2. What makes a bar that contains only chocolate different from other chocolate bars?

3. Do you think chocolate is pure? Why or why not?

• Organize the candy bars into categories.

4. Did your group choose the same categories as other groups? Could you improve your system of categories?

5. What considerations do you need to make when designing a classification system?

Classifying Substances

Take a look around you. Everything is made of matter—including your own body, the products you use, Earth, and the universe (**Figure 1**). **Matter** is anything that has mass and takes up space. Matter is made up of many different kinds of substances. Some of these substances are similar to each other, and some have obvious differences. It is these similarities and differences that allow us to classify them.

Question

Which similarities and differences among substances can be used to organize, or classify, matter into different types?

Hypothesis

If we choose certain properties, then we can classify all forms of matter.

Procedure

Part 1: Observing Properties of Matter

Materials

- apron
- rubber gloves
- safety goggles
- substance samples, e.g., chalk, tennis ball, iron nails, salt, powdered drink mix, stainless steel nuts and bolts, air, water, celery, carrot sticks, mixed nuts, flour, alcohol, sand, charcoal
- magnifier
- test tube
- 50-mL beaker
- paper

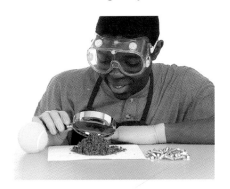

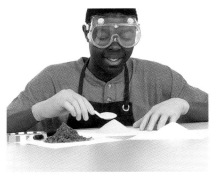

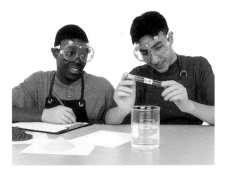

1 Make an observation table like the one below.
- **(6D)** Examine the samples that are solid, hard objects.

  ✎ (a) List all the properties you observe in your table.

2 Place a spoonful of each of the powdered solids onto a separate piece of paper.
- Use a magnifier to carefully examine each sample.

  ✎ (a) Record all the properties you observe in your table.

3 Observe the liquid and gas samples (do not remove these samples from their containers).

  ✎ (a) Record your observations in your table.

  (b) Based on all your observations, classify the different types of matter into groups.

Observations

Sample	Observations	Observations after mixing with water	Observations after mixing with other solids
?	?	?	?
?	?	?	?

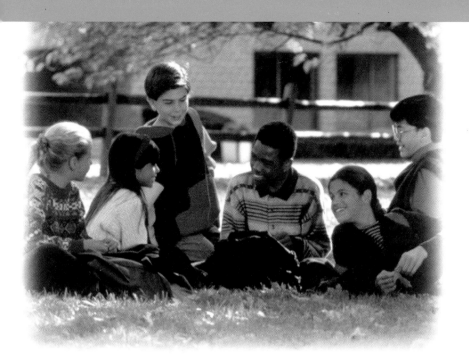

Figure 1
Matter includes all things that have mass and take up space.
There are many useful ways to categorize matter.

Part 2: Observing Properties of Mixed Samples

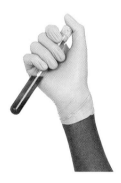

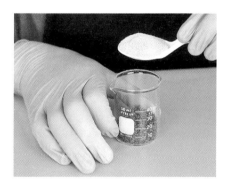

4 Place a spoonful of one of the powdered solids into a test tube. Add water to fill half the test tube.
• Put your thumb over the end of the test tube and invert it. Hold it away from your body and shake.
✎ (a) Record your observations in the third column of your table.
• Wash out the test tube and repeat step 4 with each of the powdered solids.

5 Select two of the powdered substances and mix together a spoonful of each in a beaker.
✎ (a) Record your observations in your table.
(b) Do all of the mixtures you've made fit in your original classification system? If not, change your system so all of the forms of matter you've observed can be classified.

Making Connections

1. Using your classification system, describe how you would categorize the following:
   (a) cheese and pepperoni pizza
   (b) orange juice
   (c) smoke
   (d) wood

Exploring

2. In separate containers, mix water with cocoa, gelatin powder, and ground coffee. Record your observations, and classify each mixture according to your system.

Reflecting

3. Speculate why it is helpful to classify matter.

Analysis

6 Analyze your results by answering these questions.

(a) Compare your classification system with those of your classmates.

(b) What are the similarities and differences among the different classification systems?

(c) Create a flowchart of your classification system.

Design Challenge

Think about how you could separate each mixture you made in Part 2 of this investigation so that you could have the original substances you started with. Rate each mixture as "easy to separate," "difficult to separate," or "probably cannot be separated." Explain why you rated each mixture as you did.

Pure Substances and Mixtures

In the previous investigation you looked at different substances. But why is each substance different from other substances? Why does each substance have its own properties?

The Particle Theory

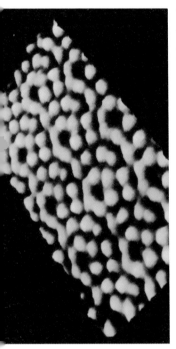

To answer these questions we need to look at the **particle theory**. The particle theory, developed over many centuries, explains that matter is made up of tiny particles with spaces between them (**Figure 1**). Particles are always moving. The more energy they have, the faster they move. The particle theory also explains that the tiny particles in matter are attracted to each other (**Figure 2**). This theory has been useful in explaining some observations about the behaviour of matter.

Figure 1
A magnified view of a thin metal foil supports the particle theory explanation that matter consists of tiny particles with spaces between them.

Different Particles, Different Substances

According to the particle theory, there are many different kinds of particles. The differences between the particles cause the substances that contain them to have different properties.

Pure Substances

A **pure substance** contains only one kind of particle throughout. There are many pure substances, but only a few can actually be found in nature! We often think of our drinking water as being pure, but this water has chemicals in it to remove bacteria, so it is actually made up of several pure substances. In nature, pure substances tend to mix together. There are exceptions; for example, diamonds are pure. They are formed deep in the mantle of Earth's crust, but they are rarely found.

Almost all of the pure substances we encounter in our lives have been made pure by human beings. Aluminum foil is pure, and so is table sugar. To obtain these substances in a pure form, we take the **raw material** that contains them, and separate out the substance we want, as shown in **Figure 3**. All samples of pure substances have the same properties whether the sample is large or small.

Figure 2

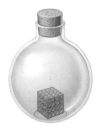

Solid
In a solid, the particles are close together and locked into a pattern. They can move, but only back and forth a little. Attractive forces hold the particles together.

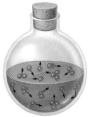

Liquid
In a liquid, the particles are slightly farther apart. Because the particles are farther apart, the attractive forces are weaker. They are able to slide past one another.

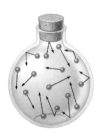

Gas
In a gas, the particles are far apart. The particles can move in any direction because the attractive forces are weakest.

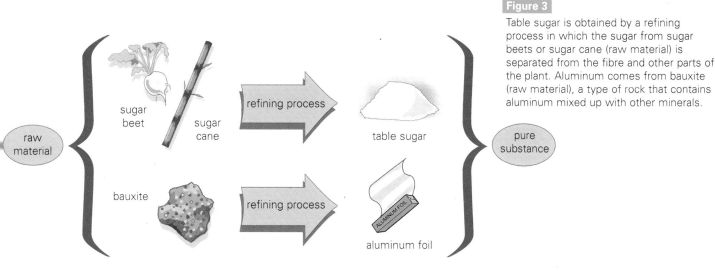

Figure 3

Table sugar is obtained by a refining process in which the sugar from sugar beets or sugar cane (raw material) is separated from the fibre and other parts of the plant. Aluminum comes from bauxite (raw material), a type of rock that contains aluminum mixed up with other minerals.

Mixtures

Almost all of the natural substances, as well as human-made and manufactured products, in the world are mixtures of pure substances. A **mixture** contains two or more pure substances, as shown in **Figure 4**. Mixtures can be any combination of solids, liquids, and gases. For example, soft drinks are a mixture that includes liquid water, solid sugar, and carbon dioxide gas. Bread is a mixture of yeast, flour, sugar, water, air, and other chemicals.

Figure 4

Most substances you will come in contact with are mixtures. Mixtures contain at least two pure substances.

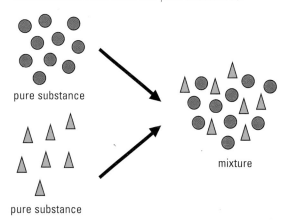

pure substance

pure substance

mixture

Try This   Is Tap Water a Solution?

- Clean two glass containers or watch glasses, ensuring that there are no spots on them.

- Mark one container T (for tap water) and the other D (for distilled water).

- With a clean medicine dropper, add 5 drops of tap water to the container marked T, and 5 drops of distilled water to the container marked D.

- Place the containers near a sunny window or a heater, and let them stand until the water evaporates.

- Hold the containers up to the light.

1. What do you notice about each container?

2. Based on your observations, is tap water a solution? Explain.

3. How would you classify the distilled water? Explain.

4. Do you think evaporation is a reliable method for separating a dissolved solid from all liquid solutions? Why or why not?

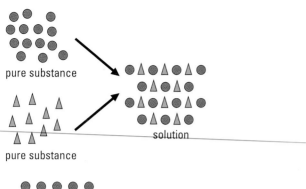

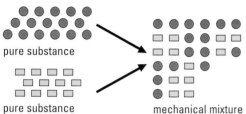

Pure substances mix to form mechanical mixtures or solutions. In a solution, the particles of the pure substances are mixed evenly so that neither original substance is visible. In a mechanical mixture, the substances do not mix evenly. Both substances are clearly visible.

Heterogeneous and Homogeneous Mixtures

In many mixtures, like concrete or granola, you can clearly see separate pieces in the mixture. Each spoonful of granola is different. If you take up a spoonful of wet concrete, it may or may not contain a pebble. This type of mixture is called a **heterogeneous mixture** (heterogeneous means "different kinds"),

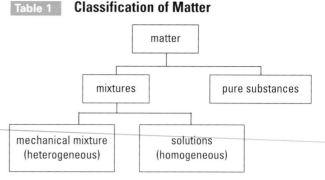

Table 1 **Classification of Matter**

because two or more substances can be seen and felt. If you take a small sample from such a mixture, it may have different properties from another sample. Another name for a heterogeneous mixture is a **mechanical mixture** (see **Figure 5**).

In a **homogeneous mixture** (homogenous means "same kind"), the particles of the pure substances mix together so completely that the mixture looks and feels as though it is made of only one substance. No matter where you sample it, or how small the sample is, the properties of this mixture are always the same. Steel, composed of iron, oxygen, and carbon, is a homogeneous mixture. No matter where you cut a steel bar, it always looks the same. When you mix a small amount of salt with water you create a homogeneous mixture. Another name for a homogeneous mixture is a **solution**. We can classify matter based on its observable properties (see **Table 1**).

Try This Mechanical Mixtures and Solutions from the Refrigerator

- Make a jelly dessert in a clear glass bowl following the package directions. When the jelly has set, observe it closely.

1. Is the jelly transparent?

2. Can you see more than one type of particle?

3. How would you classify it?

4. Is the jelly a solution?

- Try shining a flashlight through the bowl, so any fine particles will become visible.

5. What do you think now? Would you change your classification? State reasons.

- Add a tablespoon of chocolate syrup to a glass of water and stir until the syrup and water are thoroughly mixed.

6. Is the mixture homogeneous (a solution) or heterogeneous (a mechanical mixture)?

- Let the mixture stand for a while, then observe it again.

7. What do you notice?

8. Make a list of other mixtures that have similar properties to chocolate syrup and water.

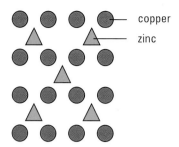

Figure 6

Brass, a decorative metal, is a solid solution in which a small amount of zinc (the solute) is dissolved in copper (the solvent) while it is molten hot. The zinc makes the brass harder than pure copper.

More About Solutions

In a solution, one substance has mixed completely, or **dissolved**, into another. Solutions can be solid, liquid, or gas. Steel, a solid solution, is made when oxygen (a gas) and carbon (a solid) dissolve into the main substance, iron. The substances that dissolve (in the case of steel, oxygen and carbon) are called the **solutes.** The substance into which they dissolve (iron) is called the **solvent.** Brass is another solid solution. The solvent in brass is copper, and the solute is zinc, as you can see in **Figure 6**.

Air, a solution of gases, consists mostly of nitrogen gas (the solvent). The gases dissolved in it include oxygen, argon, and carbon dioxide (the solutes).

Liquid solutions are formed when a solid, a liquid, or a gas dissolves in a liquid. For example, apple juice is a solution of sugar and minerals (the solutes) dissolved in water (the solvent). The oceans are a solution of many different salts dissolved in water. Another liquid solution is vinegar. Vinegar, used on French fries and salads, and for cleaning stains, is a solution that consists mostly of water (the solvent) and a small amount of liquid acetic acid (the solute).

Liquid solutions may also include dissolved gases. Pop is a sweet solution that is mostly water (the solvent), with both solid sugar and carbon dioxide gas (the solutes) dissolved in it. All solutions are homogeneous, so they look the same throughout, but liquid and gas solutions are also transparent (you can see through them). They may have a colour, however, as the solutions apple juice and tea do.

Understanding Concepts

1. **(a)** What is a pure substance? Give an example.

   (b) What is a mixture? Give an example.

2. Identify the solute and the solvent in the picture below.

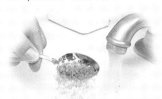

3. Describe in your own words the difference between a mechanical mixture and a solution. Include the terms homogeneous and heterogeneous in your answer.

4. Which of the following is a solution, and which is a mechanical mixture? Explain the reason for your choice.

   (a) wood   **(c)** tap water

   (b) orange juice   **(d)** loonie coin

Making Connections

5. Give an example of each of the following types of solutions (not including those already mentioned in this section):

   (a) a liquid in a liquid

   (b) a solid in a solid

   (c) a solid in a liquid

6. Make a chart and list 10 liquids found at home. Examine the contents by reading the labels on the containers.

   (a) On your chart identify the liquids that meet the definition of a solution.

   (b) For each solution, list the solvent and the solute(s) on your chart.

Design Challenge

Are the mixtures you must separate for your Challenge mechanical mixtures or solutions?

SKILLS MENU
○ Questioning　　● Conducting　　● Analyzing
● Hypothesizing　● Recording　　● Communicating
○ Planning

Filtering Mechanical Mixtures

Since most substances are mixtures, there are many situations when we want to separate the parts of a mixture. For example, you don't want to drink water that contains a mixture of soil, tiny plants and animals, and dissolved chemicals. Several techniques are available to separate mixtures. The water we drink is made safe by treating it at a water treatment plant to take out the impurities. Filtration is a technique that is frequently used in water treatment to separate particles from a mechanical mixture. Depending on the size of the particles that are being separated, the size of the mesh in the filter can be large, as in a screen, or very small, as in filter paper.

Question

Will filter paper separate all solid particles from a liquid mechanical mixture?

Hypothesis

2C **1** Write a hypothesis for this investigation.

Experimental Design

You will test whether filter paper can be used with three different mechanical mixtures.

Materials

- apron
- safety goggles
- filter paper
- milk
- water
- ground pepper
- flour
- support stand
- ring clamp
- funnel
- 350-mL beakers
- water bottle with squirt top
- stirring rod

Procedure

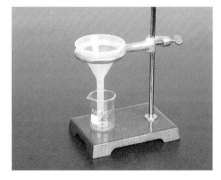

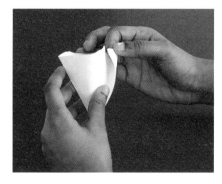

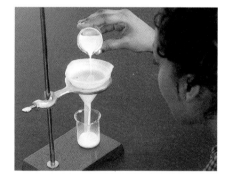

2 Set up a support stand, ring clamp, funnel, and beaker as shown above.

Wash your hands with soap and water after you complete this investigation.

3 Fold a piece of filter paper in half twice and shape it into a cone.
- Place the filter paper in the funnel.
- Squirt the paper cone with water so that it stays in place in the funnel.

4 Measure 25 mL of milk into a graduated cylinder.
- Pour the milk into the funnel.
- Wait a few moments for the liquid to pass through.

(a) Observe the filtered liquid in the beaker. How does it compare with the milk?

(b) Is there any residue left on the filter paper?

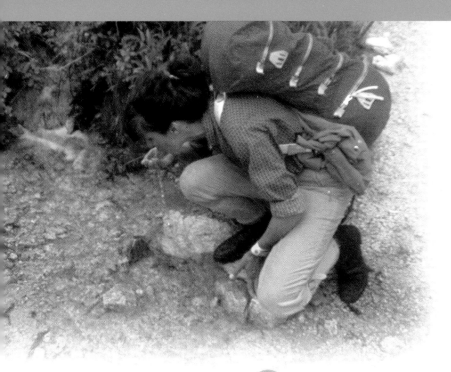

Figure 1

Water taken from a fast-moving stream will contain small particles of soil and microscopic living things. Filters can help to remove many of these particles from water. But even if water looks clear, does that mean it is safe to drink?

Design Challenge

Could you use a filter for separating materials in your Challenge? If so, what size must the mesh be? What forces will the filter have to resist? What materials should the filter be made of?

Making Connections

1. Describe how you could use kitchen utensils to separate each of the following mechanical mixtures:

   (a) sugar, toothpicks, and uncooked rice

   (b) chocolate chips, chocolate-covered peanuts, and small marshmallows

Exploring

2. Birdseed contains several types of seeds. With 250 mL (2E) of birdseed, design a procedure with your group to find out the amount of each type of seed, in units of mass or volume. With your teacher's approval, try it.

3. The screens on your windows and doors are filters that separate insects such as flies and mosquitoes from the air. Make a chart and list the different types of filters that might be found at home, at school, or in a car, as well as their purpose.

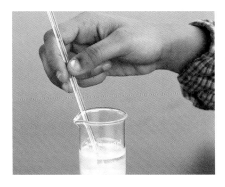

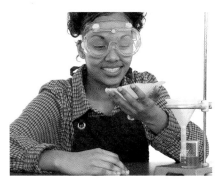

5 Remove the used filter paper and rinse the funnel with water.
- Measure out 25 mL of water in a graduated cylinder and pour it into a beaker.
- Mix 2.5 mL of flour into the beaker and stir.
- Repeat steps 2 to 4 using this mixture instead of milk.

6 Measure out 25 mL of water in a graduated cylinder and pour it into a beaker.
- Mix 2.5 mL of pepper into the beaker and stir.
- Repeat steps 2 to 4 using this mixture.

Analysis

7 Analyze your results by answering these questions.

(a) What evidence do you have that each of the liquids in this investigation is a mechanical mixture?

(b) What feature of the filter would you change to completely separate the substances in each of the mechanical mixtures?

(c) Based on your observations, was your hypothesis correct?

Are All Solvents Alike?

As you learned earlier, a solvent is a substance in which other substances, or solutes, are dissolved. Centuries ago, scientists spent much time in their laboratories experimenting with solvents. They were hoping to find one solvent that dissolved everything. Instead, they found that solvents have different abilities to dissolve different substances (**Figure 1**).

Materials
- apron
- gloves
- safety goggles
- water
- ethanol
- test tubes
- rubber stopper
- flashlight
- salt, sugar, flour, rice, bath salts, butter, candle wax, drink crystals

Question
Are the solvents water and ethanol alike?

Hypothesis

1 Read the Experimental Design and write a hypothesis that this investigation will attempt to prove.

Experimental Design
You will mix a variety of substances into both water and ethanol, and observe which ones form solutions, and which form mechanical mixtures.

 Ethanol is toxic and flammable. Do not allow it to come in contact with your skin; do not allow an open flame in the room.

Procedure

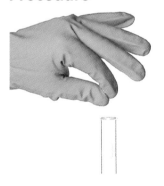

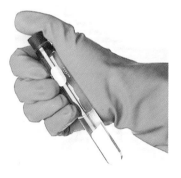

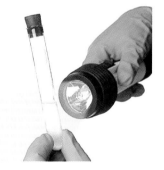

2 Pour 15 mL of water into a clean, dry test tube.
- Add a pinch of salt.

✏ (a) What happens in the test tube? Record your observations.

3 Place the rubber stopper in the test tube and shake it away from your body while you count to 5.
- Let the test tube stand for a minute or so.

✏ (a) Has any change occurred in the test tube? Record your observations.

✏ (b) Record whether the test tube contains a mechanical mixture or a solution.

4 Repeat steps 2 and 3 with each of the substances you are given, using water as the solvent. If you are not sure if a mixture is clear or cloudy, try shining a flashlight through it, so any fine particles will become visible.

(a) Which mixtures have fine particles suspended in the water? Are they solutions or mechanical mixtures?

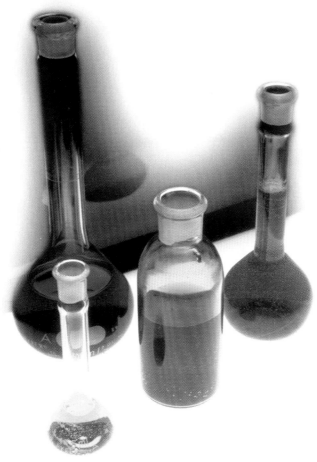

Figure 1
Different solvents have different properties. How will this affect their ability to dissolve various solutes?

Making Connections

1. Dry-cleaning machines use a liquid to dissolve and remove grease, but the liquid is expensive. What are some possible ways of reducing this expense?

2. Imagine that you have accidentally spilled perfume into a bath. The perfume contains a rare, expensive oil, which you can see floating on the bath water. What steps could you take to recover as much of the oil as possible?

Exploring

3. Oil spills that occur near shorelines are often cleaned up with the help of powerful detergents. How do you think this works?

Reflecting

4. How would you classify the mixtures in this investigation? Which mixtures are possible to separate using the filtration technique from Investigation 1.3 or the evaporation technique from the Try This in 1.2?

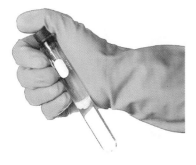

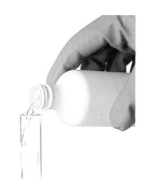

5 Dispose of the contents of the first set of test tubes, as directed by your teacher. Rinse the tubes and shake out any water.

6 Repeat steps 2, 3, and 4 using ethanol instead of water to test each of the solids you are given.

✎ (a) Record your observations.

Analysis

7 Analyze your results by answering these questions.

(a) Which substances formed a solution when mixed with:
• water?
• ethanol?

(b) Which substances formed a mechanical mixture when mixed with:
• water?
• ethanol?

(c) Write a summary paragraph to support or disagree with your hypothesis.

How Do Solutions Form?

Why do some substances mix easily to form solutions, while others do not mix at all? For instance, in the previous investigation you observed that salt mixes readily with water to form a solution, yet does not form a solution with ethanol.

The Particle Theory and Drink Crystals

To answer this question we need to revisit the particle theory. When you make a drink, you may mix together drink crystals and water. Each solid drink crystal contains billions of small particles that are tightly attracted to each other. As long as they are in their package, they will stay in their crystal form. However, when the drink crystals are mixed into water, the particles at the surface of the crystal are attracted to water particles, as shown in **Figure 1**. If the attraction to the water particles is at least as strong as to other drink crystal particles, some of the particles on the surface of the crystal will break their connections to the rest of the crystal and float off into the water. This process continues until the drink crystals break apart and mix completely, or dissolve, in the water.

If the particles of the solute are not attracted to the particles of the solvent, the two substances generally cannot form a solution.

How Do Solute and Solvent Particles Fit Together?

When the tiny particles of a solute are dissolved, or mixed completely, with the particles of a solvent such as water, the solute particles fit in the spaces between the solvent particles.

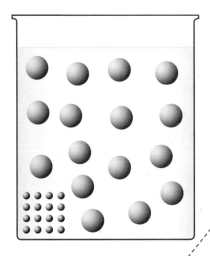

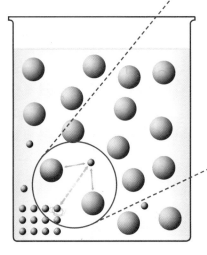

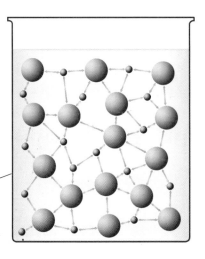

A solution occurs when all the drink particles break apart from the crystal, and mix completely with the water particles.

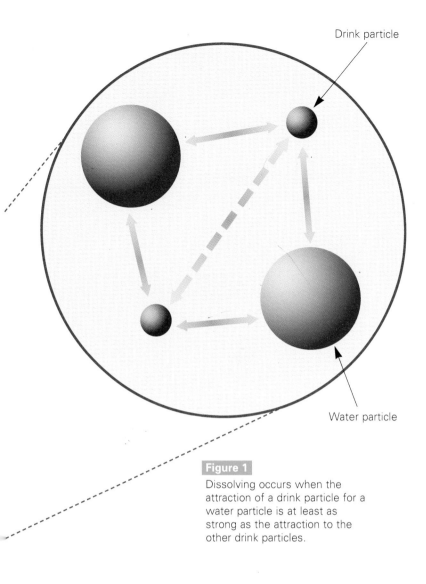

Drink particle

Water particle

Figure 1
Dissolving occurs when the attraction of a drink particle for a water particle is at least as strong as the attraction to the other drink particles.

Understanding Concepts

1. Draw and label a series of diagrams to show the sequence of events that occurs when a sugar cube is dropped into water.

(6C)

(a) How does the particle theory explain how a solute dissolves in a solvent?

(b) Based on the particle theory, why would a substance dissolve in one solvent, but not in another?

Making Connections

2. Imagine that you could take all the students in your class to the gym to help you illustrate the process of dissolving. What instructions might you give them?

3. Using what you know about particles, predict two ways you could shorten the time it takes to dissolve sugar in a drink. Explain your predictions.

Reflecting

4. Make a general statement relating the sizes of particles of substances and their combined volume when they are mixed.

Try This   A Model for a Solution

You can make a model of the solute and solvent particles in a solution. The advantage of a model is that you can observe a process that you ordinarily wouldn't be able to see.

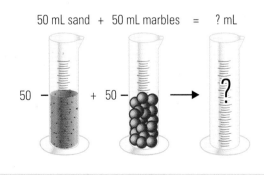

50 mL sand + 50 mL marbles = ? mL

• Half-fill a clear container with marbles and mark the level with a grease pencil or marker. Then half-fill a second, identical container with sand.

1. Predict the total volume that will result when the marbles and sand are combined.

• Carefully pour the sand into the container of marbles and shake gently.

2. How accurate was your prediction of the volume of the mixture? Explain.

3. How is the container of sand and marbles like a solution?

Flaky Baking

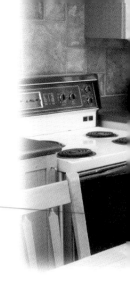

In baking, flour, fat, and water are mixed together. So why is making good pastry so difficult? The behaviour of matter is affected not only by the properties of the substance, but also by external factors such as temperature and humidity.

The main ingredients don't seem very mysterious (**Figure 1**), but getting the right mixture of these common substances remains a mystery that takes apprentice bakers years to master.

Flour and Water

The secret to flaky pastry lies in knowing how the three main ingredients work together. Flour contains many substances, including minerals and other nutrients, but the protein in the flour is pastry's "backbone." When flour mixes with water, the protein forms a substance called gluten, which gives dough strength and elasticity. But "sturdy" and "elastic" are not words you want to hear after critics have taken a bite of your pastry. What is needed is just enough strength to hold the crust together. That is why most of the steps and ingredients in a pastry recipe are designed to minimize gluten development. For example, pie crust is less likely to be tough if cake and pastry flour is used, instead of bread flour. Cake and pastry flour is 7% protein; bread flour is 12% protein.

(a) Explain how bread flour would make tougher pastry.

Fat and Flour

Liquid fat and oils do not form a water solution. Instead they will form a layer floating on water. If you force them to mix they will form a mechanical mixture, with fat forming globules in the water. It is this property that enables fat to play a major role in pastry by "waterproofing" flour particles. Small globules of vegetable shortening, lard, or butter can surround flour particles. Whenever water cannot reach the flour, gluten cannot form. When there is enough fat in the mixture, gluten forms only short strands.

(b) Why is the term "shortening" often used instead of "fat"?

(c) Why is it a good idea to add fat to the flour before adding water?

(d) What kind of mixture is dough? Explain.

Cold and Flaky

If you experiment with making pastry, you will find that cold, firm fat makes the flakiest pastry. The reason can be found in the oven.

Flaky pastry is made of many fine layers. In the oven, it is fat that separates the layers of dough. As the water in the dough turns to steam and expands, it pushes these layers of dough apart, forming the characteristic blisters or flakes of good flaky pastry. The greater the number of layers, the flakier the final pastry will be.

(e) Speculate as to why cold fat would create more layers in the dough than warm fat.

.... It's the Humidity

The dough mixture is sensitive. Even the weather has an effect!

Water holds the flour and fat together. When making pastry it is important to add only enough water until lumps of dough start to stick together. Any more water will develop extra gluten, which toughens the pastry. However, if bakers add precisely the amount of water their recipes call for, they'll find that on humid days their pastry will be tougher. Water vapour from the air becomes part of the mixture.

(f) On rainy and humid days, you should add less water than the recipe calls for. On dry days, you should add more. Speculate on what might happen to pastry dough that doesn't include enough water.

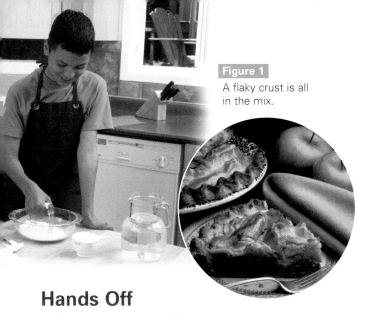

Figure 1
A flaky crust is all in the mix.

Hands Off

Too much stirring or handling of the dough toughens the pastry and also makes it less flaky. Chefs recommend you use a fork or pastry blender to mix the dough lightly, then push it into a ball with your hands.

(g) Speculate on why handling the dough too much is bad for the pastry.

Chill

Freshly mixed dough should be placed in a refrigerator for 20 min before rolling. Chilling allows the exposed flour particles to evenly absorb moisture, making the dough more uniform and easier to roll.

(h) If dough were set aside at room temperature the flour would still absorb water, but what else might happen in the dough?

Table 1	Other Pastry Ingredients
Ingredient	Function
sugars	Provides sweetness or aids yeast in producing the gas for raising dough. Sugar can tenderize dough and may help a baked product to brown.
salt	Brings out the flavours of other ingredients. Reducing or omitting salt can cause dough to rise too quickly, affecting shape and flavour.
baking soda, baking powder	Baking soda, combined with an acidic ingredient such as vinegar, lemon juice, or molasses, produces gas to raise dough. Baking powder is premixed. It contains baking soda and the right amount of acid to react with it.
eggs	Egg yolks provide uniform flavour and texture to cakes. Egg whites add air. When they are beaten, they form a froth that includes lots of air.

Understanding Concepts

1. Describe in your own words the role of each of the following dough ingredients:
    (a) flour
    (b) fat
    (c) water
    (d) salt
    (e) baking powder

2. (a) What is gluten?
    (b) What factors determine how much gluten is formed when mixing pastry ingredients?

3. Should you store shortening in a cupboard or in the refrigerator? Explain.

Exploring

4. Does noise affect rising dough or a baking cake? Could sound (2E) waves cause rising dough to collapse? Design an investigation to test the effect of sound on rising dough. Your procedure should include safety precautions. With your teacher's permission, carry out your investigation.

Other Ingredients

Recipes often call for other ingredients than the main three. Some of these are listed in **Table 1**.

Troubleshooting

An applesauce cake turned out flat, instead of airy. The recipe called for baking soda, brown sugar, and apple sauce. Both sugar and apple sauce add acid to the mix.

(i) Did the baker make an error? What could have gone wrong?

A couple from Edmonton who moved to Toronto are disappointed with their pastry, which is tougher now, at least in the summer.

(j) What would you recommend?

The Rate of Dissolving

Understanding factors that affect how quickly a substance dissolves is important to the manufacturing of medicines, dyes, and processed foods. For example, some kinds of cold relief remedies are powders that must be mixed with hot water. Scientists who work for drug companies do tests to ensure the powder dissolves quickly in hot water. Understanding how substances dissolve in other substances is an important part of their job. When you add sugar to a drink, several factors affect how quickly the sugar dissolves. Based on your experience, you probably have some idea of what these are. But have you ever tested your ideas?

Materials

- apron
- safety goggles
- beakers or clear plastic cups
- marker pen
- hot and cold water
- thermometers
- powdered sugar
- sugar cubes

Question

What factors affect how quickly a solute dissolves in a solvent?

Hypothesis

2C **1** Write a hypothesis for each variable you test in this investigation.

Experimental Design

This is a controlled experiment investigating the factors that affect the rate of dissolving. A test for one of the variables (temperature) is described in steps 6 and 7 below.

2E **2** Read steps 6 and 7. You will design and carry out tests for another two variables (particle size, stirring).

2D **3** Using sugar cubes and powdered sugar, plan a controlled procedure to test whether particle size has an effect on the rate of dissolving.

4 Plan a controlled procedure to test whether stirring has an effect on the rate of dissolving.

5 Write down the steps for your procedures and submit them to your teacher for approval.

Procedure

Part 1: Temperature

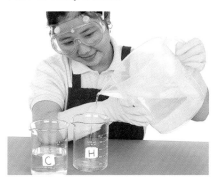

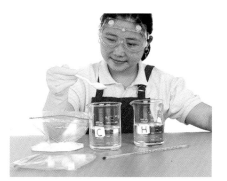

6 Mark two containers as follows: C (cold), H (hot).
- Pour cold tap water in the container marked C until it is three-quarters full.
- Pour the same amount of hot tap water into the container marked H.

✎ (a) Record the temperature of the water in each cup.

7 Add 5 mL of sugar to each cup.

(a) In which cup does the solute dissolve faster?

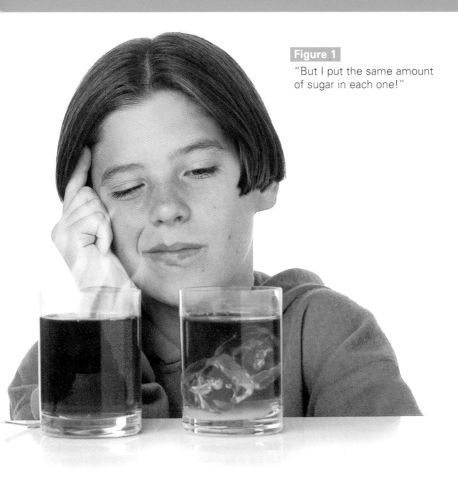

Figure 1
"But I put the same amount of sugar in each one!"

Making Connections

1. Most brands of soda pop are solutions that contain water, dissolved sugar, and dissolved carbon dioxide gas. When you remove the cap from a cold bottle of soda pop, you will hear a faint whoosh as the gas escapes. But when the cap is removed from a warm bottle, the whoosh is much louder (**Figure 2**). What effect does changing temperature and pressure have on the rate that carbon dioxide gas comes out of a soda pop bottle?

Reflecting

2. Suggest at least two procedures that you hypothesize would have no effect on the rate of dissolving. Explain why you think they would have no effect.

Parts 2 and 3: Other Factors

8 Carry out the procedures you have designed to test other factors.

Analysis

9 Analyze your results by answering these questions.

(a) List three factors that affect how quickly a solute dissolves in a solvent.

(b) What effect does each of these factors have?

(c) When testing the effect of stirring on dissolving, what was your independent variable?

(d) Explain how you controlled other variables.

(e) Use the particle theory to explain how each of the factors affects dissolving. Include a sketch in your answer.

Figure 2

Soft drinks are solutions that contain dissolved gases among other substances.

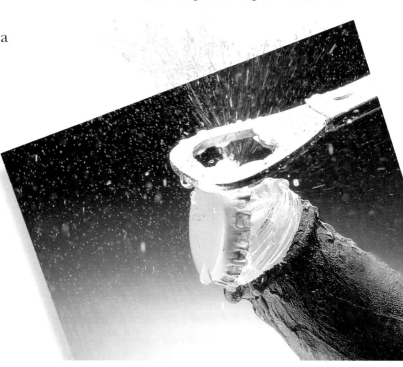

Saturated or Unsaturated?

Have you ever made a drink by dissolving flavour crystals in water and found that it tasted "watery" because you didn't add enough crystals? This happens when you don't have the right concentration of solute in the solvent. *Concentration* is the amount of solute dissolved in a given quantity of solvent or solution.

Solutions with a low concentration of solute are called **dilute solutions**. To make the flavour of your drink stronger, you must increase the concentration of the solute by adding more flavour crystals to the same amount of water. Solutions with a high amount of solute are referred to as **concentrated solutions**.

Since both dilute and concentrated solutions still contain unfilled spaces between the solvent particles (**Figure 1**), they are both **unsaturated solutions**.

The maximum amount of solute in a solution is the amount that fills all the available spaces between the solvent particles. A solution in which all the spaces are filled is a **saturated solution**. If you try to strengthen the flavour of your drink by adding still more flavour crystals to a saturated solution, the crystals will simply sink to the bottom of the glass without dissolving.

Exactly How Much Solute Can You Add?

The **solubility** of a solute is the exact amount of solute required to form a saturated solution in a particular solvent at a certain temperature.

The solubility is different for each combination of solute and solvent. The amount of solute needed to saturate a certain volume of solvent varies enormously. A solution of one substance in water, for example, may be saturated when only a little of it has been dissolved. On the other hand, a saturated solution of another substance in water may contain a lot of solute. In **Table 1** you can see that, at any temperature, the amount of sugar that will dissolve in 100 mL of water is greater than the amount of table salt, which in turn, is greater than the amount of baking soda.

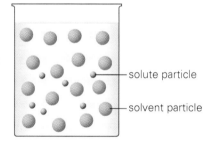

Figure 1

Dilute, concentrated, and saturated solutions

a In a dilute solution, the solute particles fill only some of the available spaces between the solvent particles.

— solute particle

— solvent particle

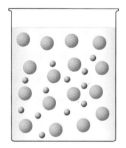

b In a concentrated solution, the solute particles fill most of the available spaces between the solvent particles.

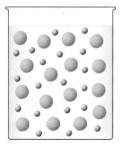

c In a saturated solution, the solute particles fill all of the available spaces between the solvent particles.

Table 1	Some Solubilities in Water		
Solute	**Temperature**		
	0°C	**20°C**	**50°C**
baking soda	6.9 g/100 mL	9.6 g/100 mL	14.5 g/100 mL
table salt	35.7 g/100 mL	36.0 g/100 mL	36.7 g/100 mL
sugar	179 g/100 mL	204 g/100 mL	260 g/100 mL

Supersaturation

With very few solid solutes, it is possible to create a solution that is more than saturated. A solution that contains more of the solute than would be found in a saturated solution is called **supersaturated**.

A supersaturated solution can be made with certain solutes by starting with a hot saturated solution at high temperature, and then allowing the solution to cool slowly. If the solution is not disturbed, all the solute may remain dissolved. Normally, as a solution cools the solute particles lose energy. This allows the attraction between a few of the solute particles to draw them together into the crystal pattern of the solid. A crystalline solid forms in the solution. In a supersaturated solution, the solute particles are not able to get into the crystal pattern.

If the container holding a supersaturated solution is struck lightly with a solid object (a spoon or a stirring rod, for example), the resulting vibrations may cause some of the solute particles to move into the crystal pattern. Immediately, the rest of the extra solute will join the crystal and fall out of solution. You can produce a similar effect by adding a seed crystal of the solute for the excess solute particles to build on (**Figure 2**).

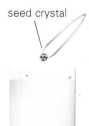

seed crystal

Figure 2

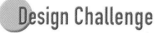

a Supersaturated solutions are rare because they are very unstable. They contain more dissolved solute than would normally occur at that temperature. Adding a seed crystal changes the nature of the solution.

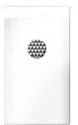

b The seed crystal begins to grow as excess solute particles are attracted to and become part of the pattern of particles in the seed crystal.

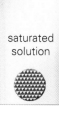

saturated solution

c All excess solute has now solidified around the seed crystal. The solution is now saturated at that temperature.

Understanding Concepts

1. Describe how you can tell the difference between a saturated solution and an unsaturated solution.

2. Is the solubility of all solutes the same?

Making Connections

3. Use the particle theory to explain why some substances do not dissolve in a particular solvent, while others do.

4. Rock candy is made by dissolving sugar in warm water to form a saturated solution, then allowing it to cool. Based on what you know about solutions, explain how the candy forms.

Design Challenge

What would you have to take into consideration designing your water purification system for Challenge 1?

Try This Comparing Solubility

- Pour 100 mL of water into each of two 400-mL beakers.

- Add 50 g of salt to one beaker and 50 g of sugar to the other.

- Stir both at the same rate.

1. Does the same amount of both solutes dissolve in the water?

2. What does this tell you about the solubility of salt and sugar in water?

Solubility and Saturation

You have already learned that the solubility of solutes in solvents is affected by temperature. But how much does solubility go up or down as the temperature rises?

Question
Are changes in the solubility of drink crystals in water predictable?

Hypothesis

2C **1** Write a hypothesis for this investigation.

Experimental Design
The solubility of drink crystals in water will be measured at different temperatures. You will be able to graph how solubility changes according to temperature.

Materials
- apron
- safety goggles
- drink crystals
- clear container
- 100-mL beaker
- 250-mL beaker
- 100-mL graduated cylinder
- water
- balance
- stirring rod
- thermometer

Procedure

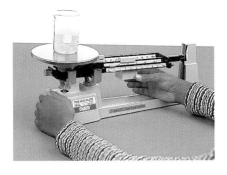

2 Measure the mass of a 100-mL beaker.

✎ (a) Record the mass of the beaker.

- Half-fill the beaker with drink crystals.
- Measure the total mass of the beaker and the crystals.

✎ (b) Record the mass of the beaker and crystals.

(c) Calculate the mass of the crystals.

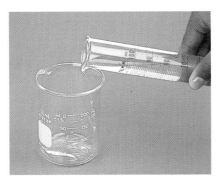

3 Fill a graduated cylinder with 100 mL of tap water.
- Pour the water into a clean 250-mL beaker.

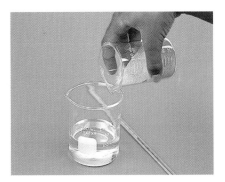

4 Slowly add crystals from the beaker to the water, stirring constantly, until no more crystals dissolve, and you see crystals starting to collect on the bottom.
- Measure the water temperature with a thermometer.

✎ (a) Record the temperature of the water.

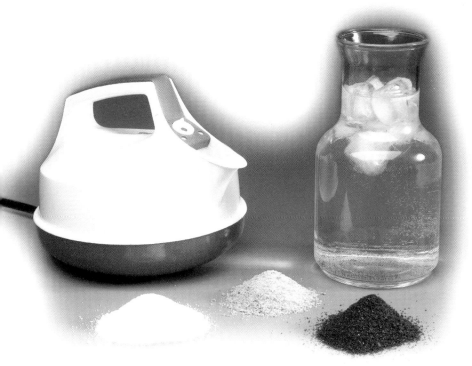

Understanding Concepts

1. If a solution is saturated at 20°C, will it also be saturated at 40°C? Explain your answer.

Making Connections

2. Suppose you mix lemon juice, sugar, and cold water to make lemonade. After stirring, there is still some undissolved sugar at the bottom of the glass.

   (a) Why didn't all the sugar dissolve?

   (b) Which type of sugar solution was formed?

   (c) What type of sugar solution would form if you heated the lemonade?

Exploring

3. Predict what will happen to a hot, saturated solution of drink crystals in water as it cools. Explain your prediction. With your teacher's permission, try it. Was your prediction correct?

Figure 1

The solubility of all solutes changes according to temperature.

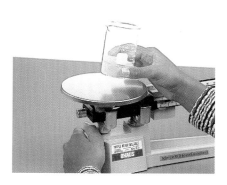

5 Measure the mass of the beaker and unused crystals and record it.

   (a) Calculate the mass of the crystals you added to the water.

   ✎ **(b)** Record the solubility of the drink crystals in water at the measured temperature, in g/100 mL.

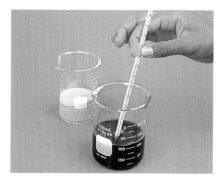

6 Repeat steps 2 to 5 using water at 3 other temperatures, using a mixture of hot and cold tap water.

   ✎ **(a)** Record the solubility of the crystals at each temperature.

Analysis

7 Analyze your results by answering these questions.

(a) How did you know when you had created a saturated solution?

(b) From your data and the data of other groups in your class, draw a graph of solubility versus temperature for drink crystals in water.

(c) Based on your graph, what happens to the solubility of drink crystals in water as the temperature of the water increases?

(d) Using your graph, predict the solubility of drink crystals in water at 80°C.

Separating Mixtures

You have learned that a mixture consists of two or more pure substances. Because each of these substances has different properties, they can be separated from each other, as shown in **Figure 1**. One of these properties may include the ability to form a solution in a particular solvent.

Question

What methods can be used to separate a heterogeneous mixture consisting of three substances?

Hypothesis

Examining the properties of the substances in a mixture will enable you to choose a technique that allows you to separate each substance from the mixture.

Experimental Design

By analyzing a mechanical mixture and studying the separation techniques illustrated in **Figure 1**, you will come up with a procedure for separating the substances.

Materials

- safety goggles
- apron
- table salt
- pepper
- sand
- sawdust
- mechanical mixture (salt, sand, and sawdust)
- iron fillings
- magnet
- 3 plastic bags
- other materials and equipment as needed

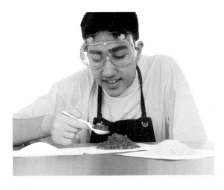

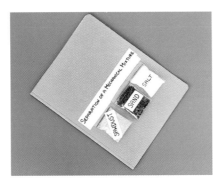

If you use a hot plate to heat a solution, the liquid may start to "spit" toward the end of the heating. Be prepared to remove the dish from the hot plate with tongs if this occurs.

1 Put on your apron and safety goggles.

2 Examine a small amount of each of the three substances in the mixture.

3 Using whatever equipment is available and your senses of sight and touch, observe and record in a table the physical properties of each substance.

4 Using what you have observed about the (2E) properties of the substances in the mixture and the information in **Figure 1**, develop a detailed procedure for separating the substances. At the end of your procedure, you must have three dry solids, each in a plastic bag. Your procedure must include labelled diagrams to illustrate how equipment will be used.

5 Submit the procedure to your teacher for approval.

Procedure

6 Once your procedure is approved, carry it out.

✎ (a) Record the appearance of your substances and mixture after each step is complete.

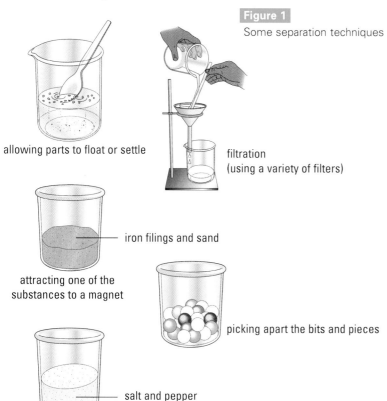

Figure 1

Some separation techniques

allowing parts to float or settle

filtration (using a variety of filters)

iron filings and sand

attracting one of the substances to a magnet

picking apart the bits and pieces

salt and pepper

dissolving one substance but not the other

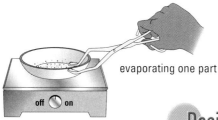

evaporating one part

off ◯ on

Design Challenge

Your Challenge requires that you separate substances in a mechanical mixture. Which of the techniques you have learned here will help you solve the Challenge?

Making Connections

1. Explain which separation techniques you might use to separate the substances in each of the mixtures below:

   (a) water, sugar, and sand

   (b) water, flour, and marbles

   (c) vegetable soup, salt, and water

   (d) water, iron filings, and soil

2. **(a)** Is there any commercial advantage to using settling instead of filtering to remove particles from a liquid? Explain.

   (b) Why isn't settling always used to separate particles suspended in a liquid?

3. Draw a flowchart to show how you would separate a mixture of iron filings, sand, salt, stones, and sawdust.

Analysis

7 Analyze your results by answering these questions.

(a) Which physical property did you use to separate the first substance from the mixture?

(b) Which physical property did you use to separate the remaining two substances in the mixture?

(c) Do you think you recovered all of each substance in the mixture? How might you improve your procedure to ensure that as much as possible of each substance is recovered?

(d) Submit a report on the ⑧ⓐ investigation that includes your observations, the procedure you used, and a description of how you would improve your procedure if you had to do the separation again.

Using Solutions of Gases

Because we can't see gases or feel them unless they move, we often forget that they exist! But we actually use many different gases in everyday life.

Air

You learned earlier that air is a solution of gases that includes nitrogen, oxygen, argon, and carbon dioxide. There are also varying amounts of water vapour and tiny amounts of several other gases. All of these gases are pure substances.

We breathe air every moment. Our lungs separate oxygen from the solution, and add carbon dioxide and water vapour. As a result, the solution of gases we breathe in is different from the solution we breathe out.

We also use air that has been compressed under high pressure for transportation and recreation (**Figure 1**).

Neon for Light

Neon is a gas that has transformed our city streets. Brightly coloured neon lights are made of glass tubes that contain neon or other gases that glow when an electric current is passed through them (**Figure 2**). Neon glows an orange colour, but by changing the colour of the glass, it is possible to make neon-filled tubes that glow red, green, or even blue. Neon and the other gases are pure substances, but neon tubes usually contain a gas solution rather than pure neon.

Gases for Surgery

Gases are an important part of surgical operations (**Figure 3**). During an operation, the patient must stay unconscious, yet still breathe. This is arranged by giving the patient a gas solution that includes oxygen and another gas, such as nitrous oxide, that causes the patient to stay unconscious. The person responsible for controlling the flow of these gases during the operation is a specialized doctor called an anesthesiologist.

Figure 4
A good, warm fire needs dry wood that will burn easily and oxgyen from the air.

Figure 1

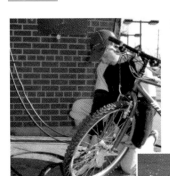

a Compressed air is used to fill bicycle and car tires for a smooth ride.

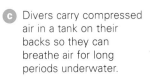

b Compressed air is also used to fill air mattresses for floating on water.

c Divers carry compressed air in a tank on their backs so they can breathe air for long periods underwater.

Figure 2
Neon light is made by passing an electric current through a glass tube that contains a gas solution that includes neon.

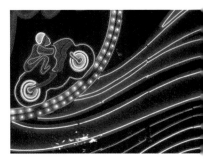

Figure 3
During surgery, the anesthesiologist controls the amounts of each gas in the solution the patient breathes. The patient must stay unconscious but also breathe normally during the operation.

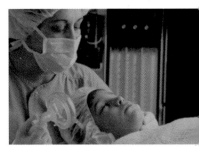

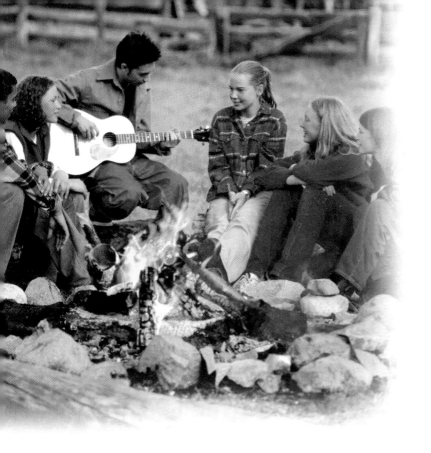

Exploring

1. Scuba divers who work at considerable depths underwater are careful not to surface too quickly to avoid a condition called the "bends" or decompression sickness.

   (a) Use a variety of print and electronic sources to research this condition.

   (b) Prepare an information pamphlet to inform scuba divers about this condition.

2. Methane gas has other surprising locations and uses. Use a variety of print and electronic sources to find out more about methane in the ocean, as an alternative fuel, and its effect on the atmosphere. Present your results as a poster that informs others about the importance of methane in our lives.

Gases for Burning

It is the oxygen in the air that allows fuels to burn. When we burn wood in fireplaces or gasoline in cars, the carbon in these fuels reacts chemically with oxygen in the air, forming carbon dioxide and water and giving off a lot of heat. This heat is used to provide warmth, cook food, or to supply energy for moving vehicles (**Figure 4**).

Sometimes the fuel itself is also a gas. For example, natural gas is piped into many homes to provide heat when it is burned in a furnace, a water heater, or a stove (**Figure 5**). Natural gas is actually a solution of several similar gases, with methane as the solvent. Like wood, oil, and coal, methane contains carbon. Natural gas is found deep underground in pockets, usually near underground oil deposits. It is believed that oil and natural gas both formed from organisms that lived millions of years ago and were buried under many layers of rock and soil. Once a gas well is drilled down through the rock to a gas pocket, the gas flows up to the surface on its own. From the surface, thousands of kilometres of pipelines bring the gas into our homes. **Figure 6** shows a pipeline.

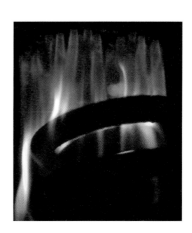

Figure 5

Natural gas is used as a fuel to heat food, water, or air.

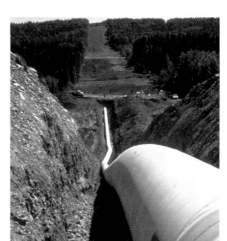

Figure 6

Extensive networks of gas pipelines extend from gas wells in western Canada to the large cities of central Canada.

Products from Raw Materials

In the beginning of this unit you learned that pure substances can be mixed together to form solutions that are liquid, gas, or solid. What are solid solutions and are they an important part of our lives (**Figure 1**)?

Most metals we use are combinations of two or more metals mixed together in a solid solution called an **alloy**. An alloy is a homogeneous mixture of a metal with other substances. Alloys allow scientists and engineers to design metals that have specific properties depending on what they are used for. Steel is formed in a process that takes iron from iron ore and carbon from coal. Usually small amounts of other metals are mixed in to give the steel different qualities. Chromium and nickel, for instance, are often added to make the steel resistant to rust, giving it the name stainless steel. Adding zinc to copper makes brass, an alloy that is stronger than copper alone and is resistant to corrosion. It is used for ornamental objects on the exterior of houses, such as house numbers and mailboxes.

The idea of making alloys is actually thousands of years old. Early civilizations discovered that if you pour a small amount of melted tin into melted copper, the tin will dissolve in the copper to form a new substance, bronze, that is much harder than either metal. Bronze was made into furniture, jewellery, tools, armour, and weapons.

Modern Alloys

We still find uses for bronze, such as in statues. However, in the past few decades metallurgists (who study metals) have experimented and come up with thousands of different alloys, each having its own special properties. Some alloys are designed to resist heat, as in **Figure 2**, others to be strong, or light, or flexible.

One important modern addition to the list of useful metals is aluminum. Aluminum is very light and is used extensively in alloys used to make automotive engines, airplanes, and bicycle frames. Aluminum helps reduce weight.

Magnesium is a metal that is even lighter than aluminum, but it is more expensive. When light weight is crucial, as in the bicycle in **Figure 3**, magnesium alloys may be used.

Ceramics

Ceramics, including pottery, bricks, cement, and glass, are made mostly from silica, and are another type of mixture. The mineral quartz is the crystalline form of silica and the source of raw materials for ceramic products. Silica particles are also often found in beach sand.

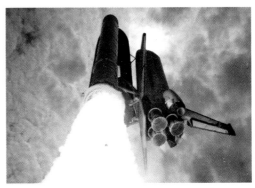

Figure 2
Rockets and jet engines are made from alloys that include tungsten, which has the highest melting point of all metals (3410°C).

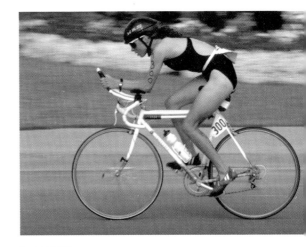

Figure 3
Bicycle frames used by racers are very light because of the magnesium dissolved in the other metals.

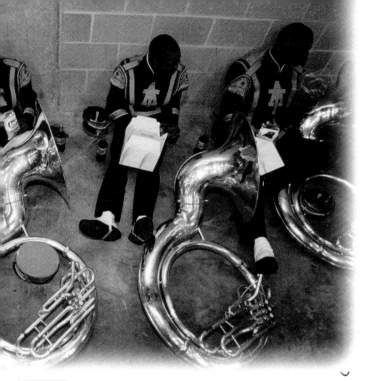

Many musical instruments, such as the saxophone, trumpet, and tuba, are made of copper and zinc mixed together to form brass.

Glass: One of the Ceramics

Glass is another type of solution—actually a supercooled liquid. The main raw material used to make glass is quartz.

Glass is a ceramic product we use daily. In the process of making glass, small amounts of limestone and potash are mixed with the silica at high temperatures, and then allowed to cool. While it is still liquid, glass can be poured onto a flat surface to form a sheet, from which we can make windows. Hot glass can also be moulded into shapes, such as vases, glasses, and bottles.

Glass Fibres

Glass can also be drawn out into fibres so thin that they are flexible but still allow light to pass through them, as shown in **Figure 4**. Thin glass fibres have revolutionized our worldwide communications systems. These optical fibres can carry thousands more signals than electrical cable made of copper wires. Optical fibres have provided the technology for the huge increase in electronic communication that has occurred in recent years.

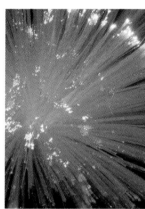

Figure 4
Optical fibres, made of glass, can carry many signals at once in the form of pulses of light. They are also used in surgical viewing instruments. Light can pass along a curved fibre, allowing the surgeon to "see around a bend."

Other Types of Ceramics

Some new types of ceramics, with different combinations of ingredients mixed in with melted silica, are able to withstand extremely high temperatures. These materials are used in the heat shields of spacecraft so that they can withstand the fiery temperatures encountered when re-entering Earth's atmosphere.

Try This — Materials with a Purpose

Purified metals, such as aluminum, nickel, or copper, and alloys, glass, ceramics, and plastic are all processed or manufactured from raw materials. Many of the products we buy have been shaped from those raw materials. In every case, the raw materials used for each item have been chosen because of their special properties.

• Look around the classroom and make a list of the objects that you see.

1. Beside each object in your list, write the materials you think it is made from.

2. Indicate if the materials are natural, such as wood, or if they have been processed, such as plastic.

3. Record some of the properties of the object and explain why the particular materials were chosen for each object.

4. Are the materials used always the best choice in each case? List any alternative materials and explain why they would be better.

Glass for Insulation

Hot, molten glass can also be spun into small glass fibres, which are sprayed with a type of glue to form thick mats. These light, fluffy mats are used as insulation in houses and other buildings to keep in their heat. As an energy-conserving measure, as shown in **Figure 5**, the use of insulation in buildings has become an important feature.

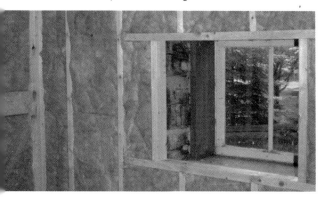

Plastics

Plastic is a modern material that we use in a huge number of products, from ice skates and toys to lawn chairs and tables (**Figure 6**). Plastic does not occur naturally. It is manufactured in a process that takes several steps, beginning with oil and gas.

Oil and Gas—the Source of Plastic

Crude oil pumped up from the Earth (**Figure 7**) is a raw material that is processed into many products, including plastic. Other products made from crude oil include gasoline, waxes, and asphalt for paving roads.

Crude oil is a mixture of many different pure substances that can be separated from each other in a refinery, as shown in **Figure 8**. The lighter substances in the crude oil are combined chemically with a pure substance from natural gas to form the many different types of synthetic materials that we call plastic.

Figure 7

Oil is the main raw material for making plastic products.

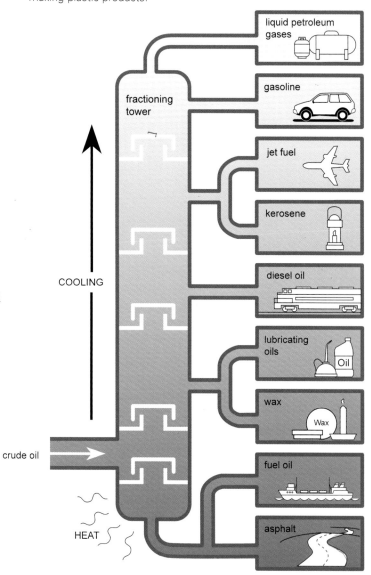

liquid petroleum gases

gasoline

jet fuel

kerosene

diesel oil

lubricating oils

wax

fuel oil

asphalt

fractioning tower

COOLING

crude oil

HEAT

Figure 6

We use plastic everywhere, for almost any activity.

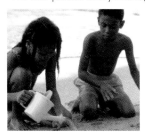
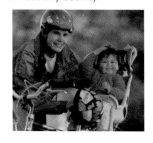
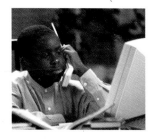

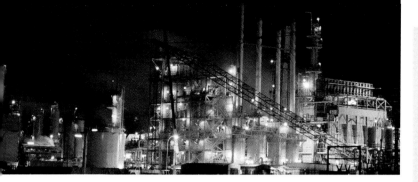

Figure 8

Crude oil is refined into many pure substances and solutions, which are then used in different manufacturing processes, for example, to make plastic and gasoline.

Materials Have Different Uses

Designers, engineers, scientists, and artists all work with materials, and must decide which material best suits the purpose that they have in mind. For example, when designing a spacecraft, engineers may have to select a different alloy or ceramic material for each part. Some parts must be extremely strong, while others must be resistant to heat, to cold, or to bending.

A glass blower may choose to add lead to glass to make a fine crystal. Glass with lead in it sparkles like a diamond when it is cut into patterns. And, of course, plastic varies widely, from the flexible form used to wrap food to the harder form used in casings, for example, around telephones and computers. We are surrounded by different materials. As consumers, we must not only make decisions about which items and which materials best suit our needs, but also about what will happen to the materials when the product is no longer useful.

Design Challenge

(a) You have learned about some finished products—plastics, glass, ceramics, metal alloys. Are any of these the best choice of material for the structures you must make for your Challenge? What other materials could you use?

(b) Different substances are used to make the various types of plastic. In the recycling Challenge, is it important to know which plastic objects can be recycled together? Are there plastics you cannot accept?

Understanding Concepts

1. Explain in your own words what an alloy is and describe its significance in the manufacturing of metallic products.

2. **(a)** What are the main raw materials used to make glass?

   (b) Which raw material is common to all ceramics?

Making Connections

3. If you had a choice of flying in a glider made of steel, or one made of a steel and manganese alloy, which would you choose? Why?

4. Many human body parts can now be replaced by artificial parts. What properties would designers and engineers need to consider when choosing the materials or substances to create an artificial limb?

Exploring

5. Soft packing beads, polar fleece jackets, and the wheels of inline skates are each made of a different type of plastic. Using electronic and print sources, research the differences between these plastics. Make a chart of the different types of plastics and what properties they have that make them suitable for the use specified.

Reflecting

6. There are many kinds of steel with many different properties. These different properties are the result of different materials added to the steel. Using electronic and print media, research how steel is made. Choose one kind of steel and create a poster illustrating how it is made, what it is made of, and how it is used.

7. "Modern products have better designs and are made of better materials than products in the past. Modern products may also have fewer environmental problems than products in the past". Do you agree with these statements? Give examples along with reasons for your answers.

Concrete for Construction

Materials
- apron
- safety gloves
- mask
- empty 1-L milk carton
- scissors
- masking tape
- plastic sheet
- concrete mix
- cement mix
- 2 containers for mixing
- mortar trowel
- water
- wire
- hook
- pail
- bathroom scales

Note that time is an important element in this investigation.

Designers and engineers must make decisions about using the best materials for a given purpose. Concrete is a material used in a variety of construction applications—buildings, dams, and sidewalks. It consists of two materials: crushed gravel and cement (**Figure 1**). The cement, when wet, is the "glue" that holds the crushed gravel together. Cement is made from clay and limestone. The gravel adds strength to the cement. But does a sidewalk need to be as strong as a dam? Is concrete as strong as cement?

Problem
How strong is cement alone compared to concrete? A construction company is preparing to build a bridge out of concrete. In order to safely ensure that the weight of people and equipment crossing the bridge will be supported, it needs to choose the stronger material of concrete or cement.

Design Brief
You will compare the strength of cement and concrete by building a cement beam and a concrete beam and comparing them.

Build

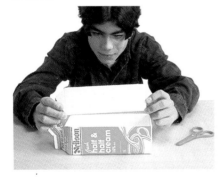

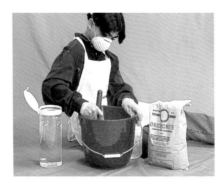

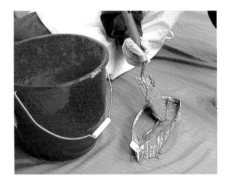

1 Seal the top of a milk carton with masking tape and lay the carton on its side.
- With scissors, cut away one side of the carton.
- With masking tape, tape the cutaway piece into the middle of the carton to form a barrier.

2 In a container, add water to 2 kg of concrete mix, stirring the concrete and water together until all the dry powder is wet.
- Use the trowel to fill one side of the milk carton with the concrete mix.

3 Repeat step 2 using cement mix instead of concrete mix, and pour this mix into the other half of the carton.
- Allow the cement and concrete to harden for two weeks, then peel away the carton.

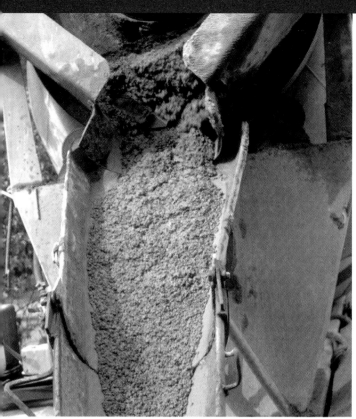

Figure 1
Concrete is a very strong material that can withstand a lot of weight without breaking. The main raw materials of concrete are gravel and cement.

Evaluate

1. Did you record any difference in the mass required to break the two beams?

2. What differences did you notice between the dry cement mix and the dry concrete mix? What differences did you notice in the beams? How do you explain the difference in strength of the two materials?

3. Which material would the construction company choose for its purpose?

Making Connections

4. Concrete varies according to how it will be used. What do you think might be the difference between the type of concrete used for dams and the type used for sidewalks?

5. The massive, 13 km Confederation Bridge links Prince Edward Island with New Brunswick. What special properties do you think would be required for the concrete in this bridge? (Hint: Consider year-round possibilities.) Research on the Internet what ingredients the engineers added to the concrete for the bridge and their purpose. *(4A)*

Exploring

6. Try making your own concrete mix by combining a different amount of gravel with the cement. Predict what will happen if you construct a beam with each different mixture and test its strength. With your teacher's permission, try it. *(3F)*

Concrete and cement mixes are corrosive. Do not handle with bare hands. Wash hands with soap and water after you complete this investigation.

Test

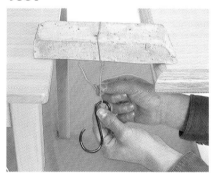

4 Place the cement beam over a gap between two tables.
- Loop a piece of wire around the middle of the beam and attach a hook.
- Suspend the pail from the hook.

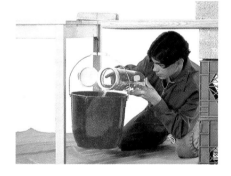

5 Gradually add sand or water to the pail until the beam breaks.
- Measure the mass of the pail and its contents.

✎ (a) Record the mass needed to break the cement beam.

6 Repeat steps 4 and 5 with the concrete beam.

Design Challenge

Would concrete be a good choice of material for any part of your Challenge?

1.14 Inquiry Investigation

SKILLS MENU
○ Questioning   ● Conducting   ● Analyzing
● Hypothesizing   ● Recording   ● Communicating
● Planning

Solvents in the Laundry

Most commercial cleaning agents are simply solvents. As you learned earlier, a substance may dissolve in one solvent but not in another. Stains are examples of substances that behave in this way. Water can dissolve some stains in clothes, but detergents are often added to dissolve many types of stains more effectively (**Figure 1**). The resulting mechanical mixture is then rinsed away.

Commercial dry cleaners also remove stains from clothes, but they use specific solvents, such as dichloromethane, that won't damage certain fabrics. From paint removers (**Figure 2**) to metal surface cleaners, industries are always on the search for better cleaning solvents.

Question

Will each of three common solvents (water, mineral spirits, and ethanol) be able to remove all of the different stains (lipstick, ballpoint ink, and felt-tip ink) from fabric?

Hypothesis

(2C) **1** Write a hypothesis for this experiment.

Experimental Design

2 Design a controlled experiment to test your hypothesis.
(2E)
* Your experimental design must include a method for placing the stained fabrics in the solvents and removing them without having your hands touch the solvents.
* Your experimental design must include a description of the variable you are testing and how you are controlling other variables.
* Your experimental design must include a description of how to dispose of the solvents safely.

3 Explain in detail how you will investigate the ability of each solvent to remove each stain.

4 Create a table for recording your data.

5 Submit your design, your procedure, and your table to your teacher for approval.

Procedure

6 Carry out your experiment in a well-ventilated room.

Materials

* safety goggles
* apron
* gloves
* labelling materials
* water
* ethanol
* mineral spirits
* graduated cylinder
* lipstick
* ballpoint pen
* felt-tip pen
* pieces of cloth
* other materials and equipment as required

 Do not touch the solvents with your hands.
* Ethanol and mineral spirits can cause damage to the skin and eyes.
* Mineral spirits are poisonous if swallowed.
* Ethanol is flammable.

Figure 1

Detergents are excellent solvents for dissolving most common stains on clothes.

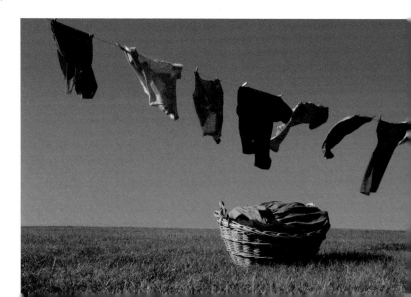

Figure 2

Turpentine is an effective solvent for cleaning (dissolving) oil-based paints from brushes. Water is effective for cleaning (dissolving) latex paints, which are made with water.

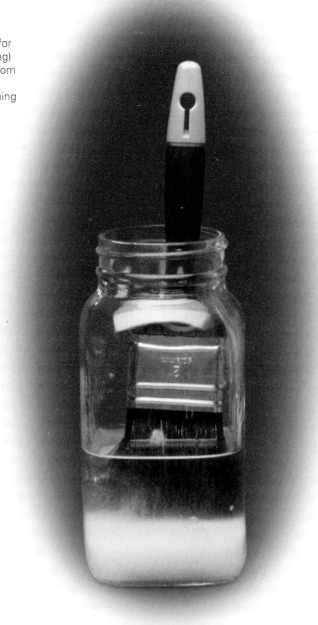

Making Connections

1. Make a list of cleaning solvents that you can find in your home. Carefully read the labels on each. Separate them into two groups: those that can be used without special precautions, and those that require special handling. What conclusion can you make about the safety of commercial solvents?

2. Imagine that you run a dry-cleaning business. You have a choice of five solvents to use. **Table 1** gives some important properties of each of them. Which solvent would you use? Explain your reasons.

Reflecting

3. Look at the properties of the given solvents in **Table 1**. What environmental concerns exist if they are disposed of by pouring them directly into the sewage system? Suggest some alternative methods of disposal.

Analysis

7 Analyze your results by answering these questions.

(a) Did any single solvent dissolve all three of the stains?

(b) If your answer to question (a) is no, which solvent removed the most stains?

(c) A good cleaning solvent must be nontoxic (not poisonous), should not be flammable, and must dissolve the stains it is being used on. Does your most effective solvent meet these criteria? Explain.

Table 1

Properties	Solvent				
	dichloromethane	turpentine	methanol	isopropanol	ethylene chloride
dissolves grease?	excellent	very good	very good	excellent	excellent
flammable?	no	yes	yes	yes	yes
toxic vapour?	yes	no	yes	no	yes

1.15

The Importance of Water

Did you know that water covers about 80% of Earth's surface? So why all the fuss about conserving water? The reason is that the oceans contain salt water that is undrinkable, and most of the rest is locked in polar ice and glaciers. That leaves less than 1% that is drinkable. But Canada, with less than 1% of the world's population, has 22% of the world's fresh water. And Ontario has 228 000 inland lakes, plus a large share of the Great Lakes. We must have more than enough.

Not quite! Water is used in more ways than you might think.

Everyday you use solutions that have water as their solvent. The tap water you drink, for instance, contains dissolved minerals that are absorbed by your body to help carry out your life functions and to strengthen your bones. You use water solutions to wash your clothes and your body. Water is also the solvent for solutions used in different industrial processes.

The problem is that people need *clean water*— water that has been filtered, processed, and purified; water they can safely drink. Tests show that our lakes and rivers contain more substances than ever that make the water less desirable for drinking. How do these substances find their way into our water supply?

Our lakes, once a source of clean water, now contain hundreds of dissolved substances. Some of the substances come from soil, rocks, and air, some from animals and plants, and some from the activities of people. Manufacturing, refining, sewage, waste disposal, farming, incinerating—these all produce substances that end up dissolved or mixed into the water that we depend on to live (**Figure 1**).

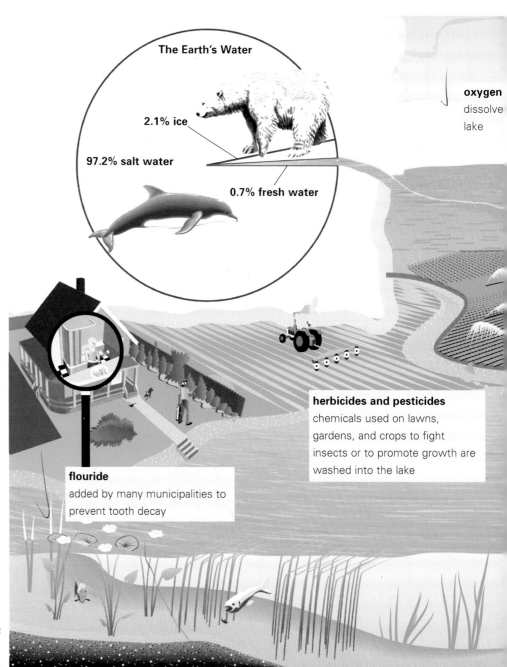

The Earth's Water

97.2% salt water

2.1% ice

0.7% fresh water

oxygen
dissolve
lake

flouride
added by many municipalities to prevent tooth decay

herbicides and pesticides
chemicals used on lawns, gardens, and crops to fight insects or to promote growth are washed into the lake

Design Challenge

A recent heavy rainfall overloaded a sewage treatment facility, causing sewage to flow into the river from which drinking water is taken. Nature can deal with such flows, if they are small. Bacteria will break down some solids, and particles of other solids will gradually fall to the bottom of the river. What can you learn from "nature's way" that will help you solve your Challenge of purifying water?

The fresh water in our lakes contains hundreds of dissolved and mixed substances. Some come from the soil, rocks, and air, some from animals and plants, and some from the activities of people. Manufacturing, refining, sewage, waste disposal, farming, incinerating— they all produce substances that either dissolve or settle in water.

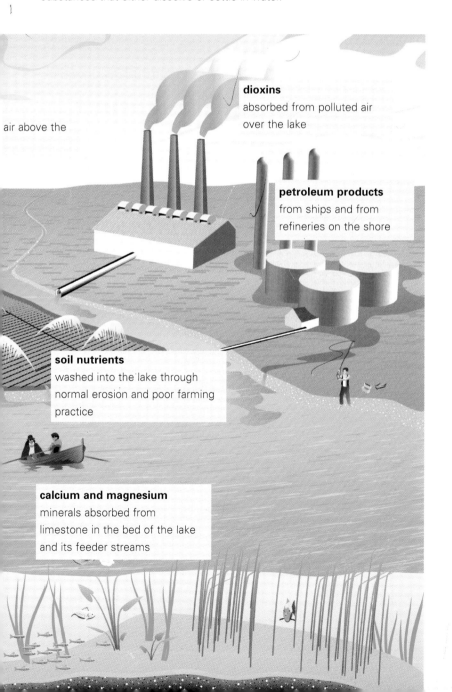

air above the

dioxins
absorbed from polluted air over the lake

petroleum products
from ships and from refineries on the shore

soil nutrients
washed into the lake through normal erosion and poor farming practice

calcium and magnesium
minerals absorbed from limestone in the bed of the lake and its feeder streams

Understanding Concepts

1. With all the fresh water in Canada, why would Canadians worry about the supply of drinking water?

2. Describe two ways in which water can be polluted from distant sources. Draw a concept map to illustrate your findings.

Making Connections

3. **(a)** How is water being used by people or animals in the picture on these pages? Make a list of the uses. Add any other uses of water that you can think of.

   (b) Put a star (*) beside each use of water that you think involves the addition of substances to the water. If you know the names of the substances, write them down beside the use.

4. Suggest some strategies for conserving water in the following places:

   (a) bathroom

   (b) kitchen

   (c) outdoors

Exploring

5. Water is easy to waste. Place a plastic measuring cup under a slowly dripping tap, either at school or in your home. Measure the time it takes to fill the cup. How much water is lost in one hour by a leaky tap? in one day? in one month?

Reflecting

6. Often liquid wastes are disposed of by pouring them down the drain. What problems can be caused by this practice? What problems are caused by industries and municipalities that dump pollutants directly into lakes and rivers?

Testing Water Quality

Clean drinking water is essential for human survival. It must be clear and free of dangerous living things and chemical poisons. For aquatic animals such as fish, water must include enough dissolved oxygen for breathing. Mostly, though, clean water is defined by what it doesn't contain. There are tests we can do to show what is in the water we drink or swim in.

Dissolved Oxygen

The amount of oxygen dissolved in water is one of the most important indicators of water quality, since oxygen is necessary for aquatic organisms to live.

Oxygen in air is able to pass from the air and dissolve into surface water. Oxygen is also produced in the water by aquatic plants. In the process of converting the energy of the sun, water, and carbon dioxide into food, plants release oxygen as waste. At night, though, aquatic plants consume dissolved oxygen and release carbon dioxide. But oxygen is also consumed by animals and bacteria in the water, as you can see in **Figure 1**.

Most aquatic organisms require a dissolved oxygen concentration of 5 to 6 parts per million (ppm) for normal growth and activity. Levels below 3 ppm are stressful for most aquatic organisms, and levels below 2 ppm are too low for fish populations to survive.

Acidity

Most water in nature contains dissolved substances that make it slightly acidic or, the opposite, slightly alkaline. Strong acids and strong bases are dangerous to living things, as both are corrosive. **Figure 2** shows the **pH scale**, which is used to classify how acidic or alkaline a solution is.

A healthy lake typically has a pH of about 8, which is slightly alkaline. Lakes that receive a lot of acid from rain or snow may end up with a pH of 4 or 5, which is acidic. In water that is acidic it is difficult for certain species of fish to survive. However, many lakes are surrounded by rocks that naturally neutralize the acid, as you can see in **Figure 3**.

You can test how acidic or alkaline a water sample is with specially coated "pH paper" that changes colour. Each colour corresponds to a pH number.

Figure 2

The pH scale ranges from 0 (strongly acidic) to 14 (strongly alkaline). Solutions at both ends of the scale are highly corrosive. The middle of the scale, a pH of 7, is neither acidic nor alkaline, so it is described as neutral. Pure water is neutral—it has a pH of 7.

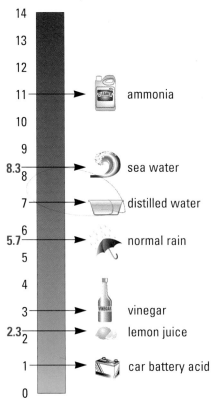

- 14
- 13
- 12
- 11 — ammonia
- 10
- 9
- 8.3 / 8 — sea water
- 7 — distilled water
- 6
- 5.7 — normal rain
- 5
- 4
- 3 — vinegar
- 2.3 / 2 — lemon juice
- 1 — car battery acid
- 0

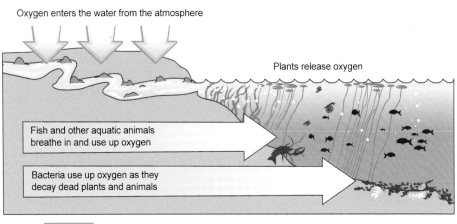

Oxygen enters the water from the atmosphere

Plants release oxygen

Fish and other aquatic animals breathe in and use up oxygen

Bacteria use up oxygen as they decay dead plants and animals

Figure 1

Oxygen is vital to living things. In a lake, there must be a balance between oxygen added and oxygen used.

Turbidity

Small solid particles are often suspended (floating) in water. These particles make the water cloudy. **Turbidity** is a measure of how cloudy water is. If water contains large amounts of suspended solids, the water will be so cloudy that it blocks sunlight from reaching aquatic plants. Without sunlight, the plants will die. Suspended solids can be caused by soil erosion, wastes from animals and plants, human waste, and waste from industry.

Special meters, using light and a light detector, can be used to measure turbidity.

Hardness

Water that contains small amounts of dissolved minerals is called **soft water**. Rain water is the best example of natural soft water.

Most water in nature contains a variety of dissolved substances. Water that contains relatively high amounts of dissolved calcium, magnesium, or sulfur is called **hard water**. Hard water is difficult to clean with, as soap does not form a lather in it. Hard water containing dissolved sulfur may have an unpleasant taste.

The dissolved substances come from the soil and rock that water passes over or through. For example, rain water that ends up in a stream that flows over limestone will dissolve calcium from the rock.

Design Challenge

In the water purification Challenge, you must propose some tests to measure the safety of the water. Which of the tests of water quality mentioned here should you include? Would you need others?

Understanding Concepts

1. Make a chart that lists four important measures of the quality of water. Note how each is important to our survival and quality of life.

2. **(a)** Describe the cycle of oxygen in a lake.

   (b) Predict what can occur if any part of the cycle is disrupted.

Making Connections

3. Imagine that people start pumping sewage into the stream that flows into the lake in **Figure 1**. Sewage water contains many small suspended solid particles. Explain what effects you would expect to see on:

   (a) the turbidity of the lake

   (b) the oxygen content of the lake

   (c) plant and animal life in the lake

Exploring

4. Using electronic and print sources, research how hardness is eliminated from water, either during the water purification process or by consumers before they use it. Prepare a chart listing the different techniques.

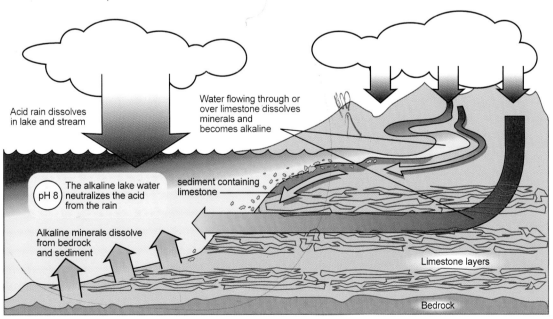

Acid rain dissolves in lake and stream

Water flowing through or over limestone dissolves minerals and becomes alkaline

pH 8 The alkaline lake water neutralizes the acid from the rain

sediment containing limestone

Alkaline minerals dissolve from bedrock and sediment

Limestone layers

Bedrock

Figure 3

In some lakes, naturally occurring alkaline substances, such as limestone, help to neutralize the acid in rain and maintain the pH at about 8.

1.17 Inquiry Investigation

SKILLS MENU
- Questioning
- Conducting
- Analyzing
- Hypothesizing
- Recording
- Communicating
- Planning

How Hard Is the Water?

Hard water forms when certain substances, such as calcium and magnesium, dissolve in it, as shown in **Figure 1**. One of the properties of hard water is that soap does not lather very well in it. However, hard water tastes better, unless it contains dissolved sulfur, and is better for you because of its mineral content.

Materials
- apron
- safety goggles
- distilled water
- 1-L container
- liquid soap
- 5-mL spoon
- ruler
- tap water
- Epsom salts

Question

2B **1** Read this investigation. What question is it attempting to answer?

Hypothesis

2C **2** Create a hypothesis for this investigation.

Experimental Design

After adding known amounts of magnesium sulfate (also called Epsom salts) to water, you will measure changes in the amount of lather produced.

Procedure

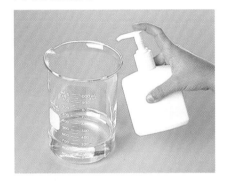 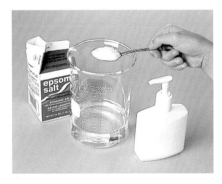 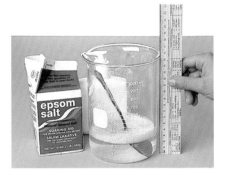

3 Place 250 mL of distilled water in a 1-L container.
- Add 2 drops of liquid soap and stir thoroughly.
- Quickly measure the maximum height of the layer of suds on the surface.

✎ (a) Record the height of the layer of suds.

4 Thoroughly rinse and dry the container before refilling it with another 250 mL of distilled water.
- Stir in 5 mL of Epsom salt crystals until they have all dissolved.
- Add 2 drops of liquid soap, stir thoroughly, and measure the height of the suds.

✎ (a) Record the maximum height of the layer of suds. Are the suds higher or lower than in step 1?

5 Repeat step 3 with fresh distilled water and 10 mL of Epsom salts.

✎ (a) Record the maximum height of the layer of suds.

SKILLS HANDBOOK: 2B Asking a Question 2C Predicting and Hypothesizing

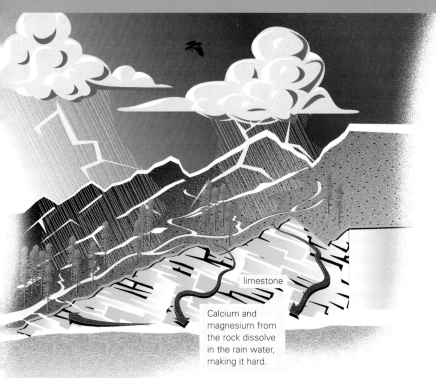

limestone

Calcium and
magnesium from
the rock dissolve
in the rain water,
making it hard.

Figure 1

Rain water, which is naturally soft, becomes hard as it runs over and through rocks and soil.

Making Connections

1. Most manufacturers of hair shampoo say that their product is not affected by the hardness of water. How could you prove or disprove this claim? Design a procedure and, with your teacher's permission, carry it out.

   (a) Based on your observations, what do you suspect is different in the ingredients of liquid soap and shampoo? Explain. Check the labels on some containers to verify your answer.

Exploring

2. Design a procedure to compare the hardness of local
   (3F) water samples from the school fountain, your home, a local stream or river, rain water, etc. You can use the graph you created in this investigation to compare the samples. Have your procedure approved by your teacher before you do any testing.

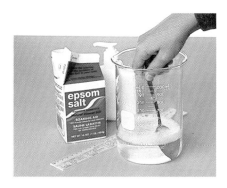

6 Continue this process, adding an additional 5 mL of Epsom salts each time, until no suds appear on the surface of the water, even after thorough stirring. Clean up any spills immediately.

✎ (a) Record the maximum height of the suds each time.

(b) Describe the final contents of the beaker.

Analysis

7 Analyze your results by answering these questions.

(a) Use your data to draw a graph
(7C) comparing the height of the layer of suds with the amount of Epsom salts added.

(b) Based on your graph, explain the relationship between the height of the lather and the amount of Epsom salts you added to your solution.

(c) What effect does Epsom salts have on water?

(d) Describe two observable characteristics of hard water.

Household Hazardous Waste

Do you contribute to water pollution like the people shown in **Figure 1**? You may not think so, but we all use many solvents and solutions at home because they help with cleaning, polishing, painting, and other activities. These **hazardous products** often require special handling and storage because they are dangerous to human health or to the environment. Labels on these products indicate how they are dangerous, as shown in **Figure 2**.

A second type of labelling, shown in **Figure 3**, gives detailed information on the safe handling of a much wider variety of chemical products. These are often found in the workplace, as well as in schools.

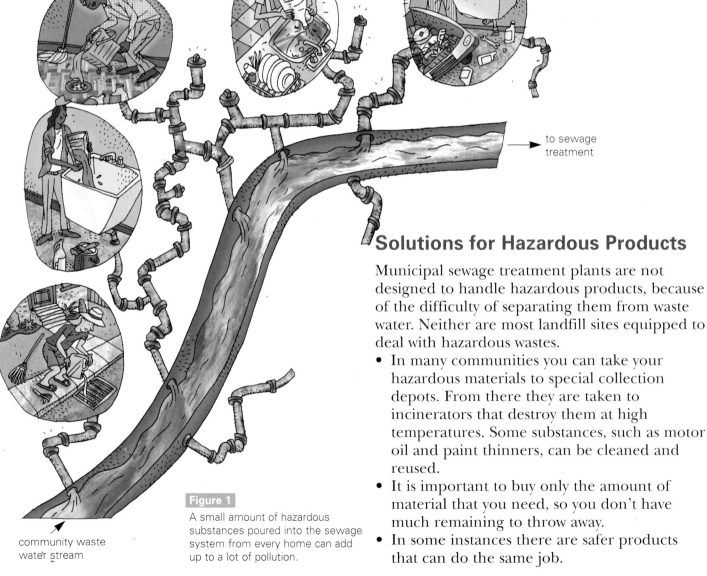

to sewage treatment

Solutions for Hazardous Products

Municipal sewage treatment plants are not designed to handle hazardous products, because of the difficulty of separating them from waste water. Neither are most landfill sites equipped to deal with hazardous wastes.

- In many communities you can take your hazardous materials to special collection depots. From there they are taken to incinerators that destroy them at high temperatures. Some substances, such as motor oil and paint thinners, can be cleaned and reused.
- It is important to buy only the amount of material that you need, so you don't have much remaining to throw away.
- In some instances there are safer products that can do the same job.

Figure 1

A small amount of hazardous substances poured into the sewage system from every home can add up to a lot of pollution.

community waste water stream

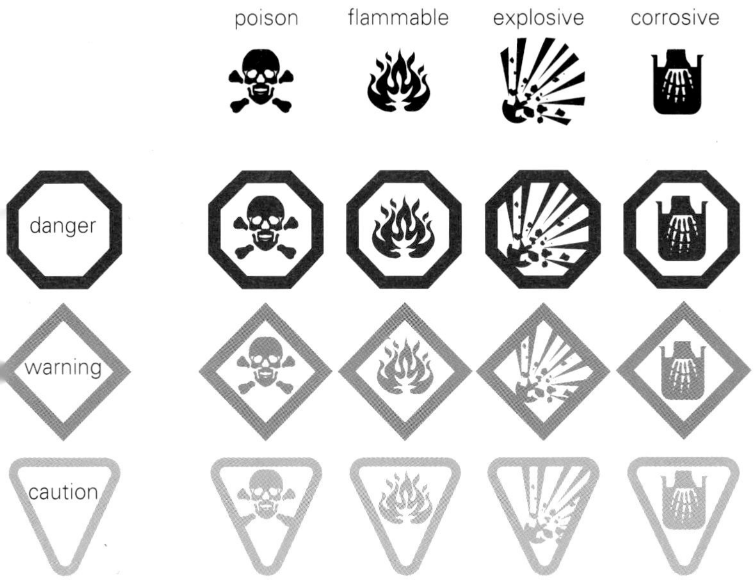

poison   flammable   explosive   corrosive

danger

warning

caution

Figure 2

Government regulations require that hazardous household products must be marked with warning symbols that indicate why, and to what degree, a product is dangerous.

 compressed gas

 dangerously reactive material

 oxidizing material

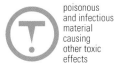 poisonous and infectious material causing immediate and serious toxic effects

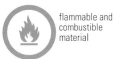 flammable and combustible material

 biohazardous infectious material

 corrosive material

poisonous and infectious material causing other toxic effects

Figure 3

Labels from the Workplace Hazardous Materials Information System (**WHMIS**). Before using any products, always read the label to check how to handle the product safely.

Understanding Concepts

1. What does the term "hazardous product" mean?

Making Connections

2. If methods of hazardous waste disposal are inadequate in your community, as a class, prepare recommendations on how disposal methods could be improved and forward them to local officials.

Reflecting

3. Some people believe that one way to solve pollution is to flush poisonous chemicals down the drain. What would you tell them?

Design Challenge

A recycling program may gather containers that hold hazardous products. How can you make the process safe for environment workers?

Try This — How Is Waste Disposed of in Your Community?

Everyone has different types of hazardous wastes in their homes. Are they being disposed of correctly?

- Create a list of hazardous products in your home. Do not open containers. Check each room, including the garage and bathroom. Beside each item, indicate whether it belongs in one of the four categories of household hazards listed in **Figure 2**.

1. What have you and your family been doing with your "almost empty" containers of hazardous waste?

- Find out how hazardous wastes are collected and disposed of in your community.

2. How do you dispose of the products listed?

(4A) **3.** Prepare an action plan for your family to dispose of hazardous waste.

Cleaning Up Our Water

You've learned that many substances dissolve in water. Unfortunately, this has resulted in pollution of many of our water systems, as people dump waste into lakes and streams.

The major source of water in Ontario, the Great Lakes, is the dumping ground for many pollutants from both sides of the border. This has been a problem for decades, as many Canadian and American cities and their industries are located on the shores of the Great Lakes. Thunder Bay, Sault Ste. Marie, Chicago, Windsor, Detroit, Buffalo, Hamilton... the list is long.

About 5800 t of pollutants are added each year. Most of the industrial waste is added to Lake Erie (40%) and Lake Michigan (28%). Less of the total is dumped into Lake Ontario (19%), and the least is added to Lake Superior (7%) and Lake Huron (6%).

Measuring the Problem

Scientists on both sides of the border are trying to learn more about each of the vast amount of chemicals that has been dumped or washed into the huge chemical solution that fills the Great Lakes. Of course, that chemical solution is also the source of drinking water for millions of people. There are many questions that these scientists must answer. For example, many chemicals are dangerous only when they reach a certain concentration. But what is the dangerous concentration for each chemical? What are the sources of the chemicals? How can we reduce the amount of these chemicals that enter the lakes?

This research, along with increasing public awareness, is gradually resulting in a reduction in the amount of waste being dumped into the Great Lakes (**Figure 1**). Although there have been significant reductions in the amounts of municipal and industrial waste being dumped into the Great Lakes, many polluters still remain.

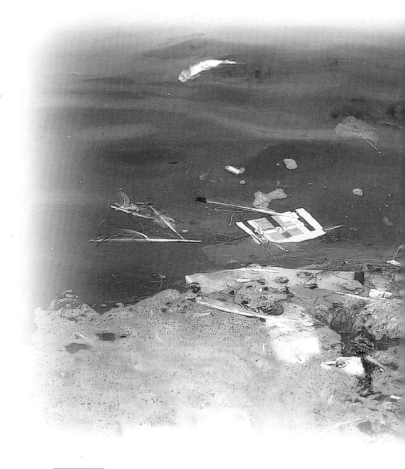

Figure 1

Pollution created by industry and our activities flows into the Great Lakes. How far should we go in reducing that flow?

Cleaning Up the Great Lakes ⑧ⅅ

Statement

The Great Lakes have been a dumping ground for both industrial and municipal (human) pollutants for hundreds of years. With adequate treatment, water from the Great Lakes still remains safe for human consumption. Appeals to reduce or eliminate pollutants at their source are often countered with arguments about the economic consequences of such initiatives. Can we continue to move at the present pace of reduction and still be assured of a safe source of drinking water in the next millennium and beyond?

Point

- Companies and cities should be permitted to dump some waste into the Great Lakes. Since the volume of water in the lakes is so large, the waste will be diluted to safe concentrations.
- The cost of waste treatment is high. If companies based around the Great Lakes are forced to spend more money on pollution control than other companies located elsewhere, products from the Great Lakes area will cost more. This could mean lost sales and lost jobs.

Counterpoint

- Even a small amount of some pollutants can cause serious effects. As the pollutants accumulate through the food chain, the concentration for humans, at the end of the chain, can become high enough to be poisonous.
- Living things depend on clean water. If the water in the Great Lakes is polluted, all living things suffer, including people. People can find other jobs, but damage to health and the environment is difficult to fix.

What Do You Think?

- Consider the statement and the points and counterpoints. Discuss. What other points and counterpoints can you think of?
- Research the issue for both sides, using newspapers, a library periodical index, a CD-ROM directory, or the Internet for information on Great Lakes water pollution.
- Form a group to represent one side of the issue. Others in your class will form a group to represent the other side.
- Conduct a debate defending each group's position.

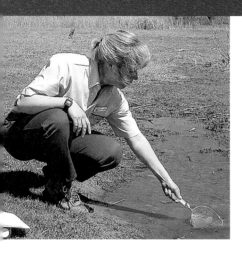

Wetlands Preservation

"Hip waders, binoculars, compass, and bug spray are some of the tools of my trade. My name is Joanna John and I am a wetlands specialist with the Upper Thames River Conservation Authority.

"Wetlands are more than just a haven for wildlife. Other benefits, such as improving water quality, decreasing downstream flooding, increasing flow in a drought, and controlling soil erosion, are also important.

"I spend a lot of time in the Thames River watershed carrying out evaluations of the wetlands. In the field, I take water samples and study the direction of water movement, make lists of plants and animals that live there, look for rare and endangered species, and note any disturbances by people.

"I work with the staff of the conservation authority and a variety of community groups and individuals to develop management plans for the wetlands. I also conduct hikes and prepare educational materials about the importance of wetlands."

An Artificial Wetland

Sewage treatment plants generally do not have the capability of removing household hazardous waste from sewage. Some cities are beginning to look to nature, specifically wetlands, to see how nature cleans water.

Based on what Joanna and her colleagues have learned about the wetlands in the Thames River watershed, engineers working for the City of London in Ontario have created Mornington Pond. Although it looks like a natural wetland, as you can see in **Figure 1**, it is a carefully designed system for controlling and purifying the huge amounts of water that collect during a storm, when the city's sewage system would normally become overloaded.

Mornington Pond is actually a series of ponds. The ponds hold and clean storm water until water flow to the sewage treatment plant returns to normal, and water levels in the river go down. The water is then gradually released into the Thames River in the same way that treated water from the sewage plant is released.

As water collects in the ponds, heavier sediment particles, often carrying contaminants, sink to the bottom, where they are periodically removed. More than 1000 native plant species planted in the ponds help purify the water by absorbing dissolved substances and controlling erosion in the same way that a natural wetland functions.

Mornington Pond is an environmentally friendly, cost-effective way of purifying water. So far, it has cost $3 million less than a traditional water treatment facility.

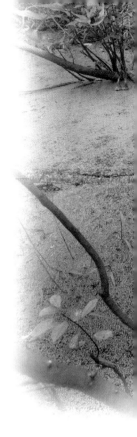

Figure 1

Mornington Pond is an artificial wetland, created by the City of London. Wetlands are rich environments, formed in areas where water drains slowly.

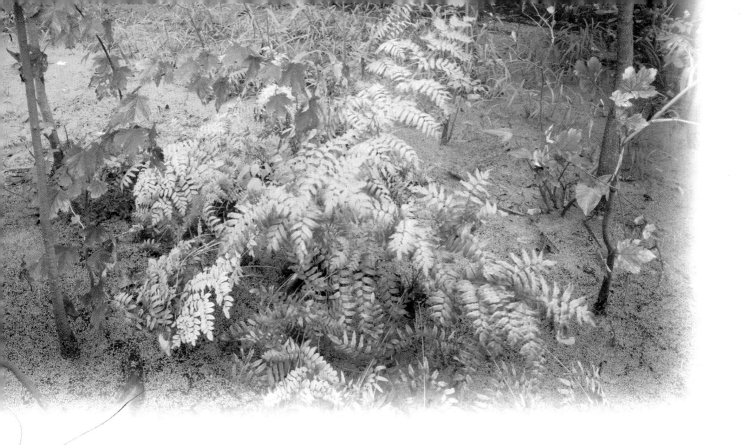

Try This — Round Table—Wetlands or a Mall? ⑧Ⓓ

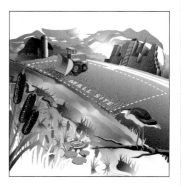

In your community, a developer, a local realtor, and the chamber of commerce are proposing to develop a new shopping mall. The mall promises to create 350 temporary construction jobs the first year, followed by 500 permanent jobs in various mall stores.

The proposed site for the new mall includes part of a wetlands area where many plants and animals live. The wetlands have also reduced flooding in the area over the years. The land is privately owned.

- List five arguments that might be used to justify moving ahead with the project as outlined.

- List five arguments that might be put forward to oppose the development.

- Decide which of the 10 arguments is the strongest and prepare to support the argument in a round table discussion. You may wish to contact local resource people while doing your research.

- Present your information and position at the round table, individually or as part of a "pro" or "con" group.

1. Did your views change during research and discussion of this issue? Explain.

2. Based on your research and the round table discussion, list the factors that are critical for deciding whether a wetland or other habitat should be destroyed when creating a new development.

3. Consider "sustainability." What implications would there be on the environment, the economy, society?

Water Additives

You have discovered that there are many substances dissolved in fresh water. After learning about water pollution, you may be wondering if all substances in the water are unsafe. In fact, some substances are beneficial. Iron, for example, is found naturally in water that flows over limestone, and is a key substance in hemoglobin, which carries oxygen in your blood.

Chlorine and Our Water

Water treatment plants, like the one in **Figure 1**, deliberately add substances to drinking water, taking advantage of its dissolving properties. Chlorine is dissolved in both drinking water and swimming pools for the same reason—to destroy bacteria. In the past, bacteria-containing water killed millions of people by causing diseases such as cholera. Chlorine is added to water supplies to eliminate such bacteria.

Most people never give chlorinated water a thought. However, scientific studies are showing a link between chlorinated drinking water and a variety of health effects. For example, chlorinated water may destroy some of the bacteria in our intestines that help us digest our food. Also, excessive amounts of chlorine in swimming pools can aggravate asthma in children.

Fluoride and Our Water

Another chemical added to drinking water to protect teeth is a compound that contains fluoride. Several studies have indicated that water fluoridation is a safe and cost-effective means of reducing tooth decay, as shown in **Figure 2**. For residents of communities that don't have water fluoridation, the alternative is regular visits to a dentist for fluoride rinses.

Since there is an alternative to fluoridating all of our drinking water, some groups feel that if there is a slight chance that fluoride might be harmful, then it should not be added to community water supplies. For example, some research suggests that long-term use of flouride may be slowly destroying our bones, teeth, and general health. Too much flouride can actually weaken teeth, making them porous and easily stained. It turns out that fish and other aquatic life don't react well to the addition of fluoride at higher-than-recommended levels.

Should we continue to add fluoride and chlorine to drinking water? Are there safer alternatives? If we continue, what is the minimum amount of these substances that we can add? Scientifically aware citizens must ask such questions to encourage study and ensure that responsible decisions will be made.

Figure 1

Many municipalities have water treatment plants where solids and dissolved substances are removed from the water to make it drinkable. These plants also add chemicals for health reasons.

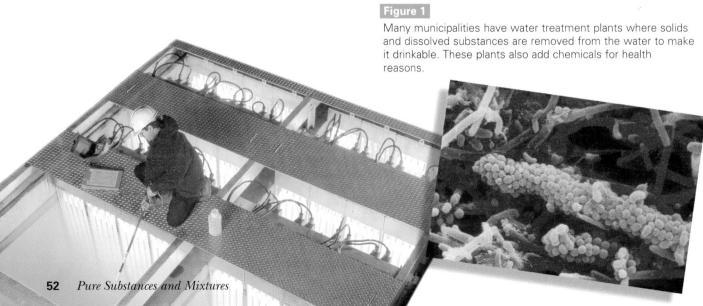

Figure 2
The bacteria that live in our mouths can be a threat to teeth.

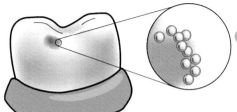

a Bacteria that feed on sugar in the mouth produce acids.

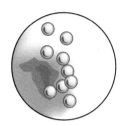

b The acid produced by the bacteria eats through tooth enamel.

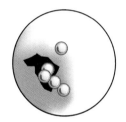

c Bacteria enter the tooth through the hole in the enamel and infect the tooth.

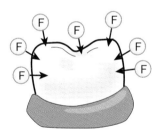

d Fluoride compounds dissolved in water enter the tooth enamel and make it stronger.

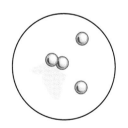

e The tougher enamel resists bacterial acid.

Understanding Concepts

1. What is one benefit and one drawback of dissolved chlorine in water?

2. Describe in your own words what is meant by fluoridation and chlorination.

3. Draw a comic strip describing the life of a bacteria on your tooth.

4. State one risk in using unchlorinated drinking water.

Making Connections

5. A thirsty hiker finds a stream in the wilderness. She has special water purification tablets in her pack but decides not to use them, since there are no houses or industries in the area. Is she right to drink the water untreated? Give your reasons.

Exploring

6. Travellers to remote parts of the world often carry small kits with them that purify water. Find out how one of these works. Where else do you think similar types of water purifiers might be useful?

7. Using electronic and print sources, research the advantages and disadvantages of adding flouride to our drinking water. Present your report to the class.

Design Challenge

How large are bacteria? Will your design for purifying water remove them?

Design Challenge

Design and Build a System That Separates or Purifies Materials

Reusing and recycling all sorts of substances and products, both liquid and solid, has become ever more important as our growing population uses more of Earth's resources and creates more garbage. Our mineral resources are limited, and so is our supply of fresh, clean drinking water. Purifying our water and separating different materials for reuse requires many types of technology.

1 A Water Purification System

Problem Situation

Although people in cities have access to purified water, those who live in rural and more remote areas may take their water from lakes and rivers, where the water is often murky due to particles mixed in it.

Design Brief

- Design and build a filtering system that removes solid particles from water.

Design Criteria

- The device must be able to remove microscopic particles from the water (verified with a microscope).
- The water must move through the filtering system under pressure.
- Additional tests must be outlined for establishing the safety of the water for drinking.

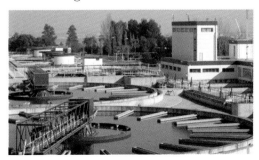

Figure 1

Water is purified for drinking. The first step in this process is to improve the clarity of the water.

2 A Recycling System for Plastic, Glass, Metal, and Paper

Problem Situation

Although many people separate the different types of recyclable materials before putting them out on the curb, recycling companies must separate the substances more accurately before they can be processed into new materials.

Design Brief

- Design a system in which a mixture of plastic, glass, metal, and paper items are separated from each other.

Design Criteria

- Each component (plastic, glass, metal, paper) must be removed from the mixture in a set sequence.
- The separation processes must be safe and efficient.
- A flow chart outlining the system must accompany the model.

Figure 2

All the materials in this yard can be recycled, but they must first be separated from one another.

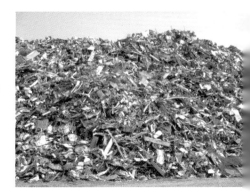

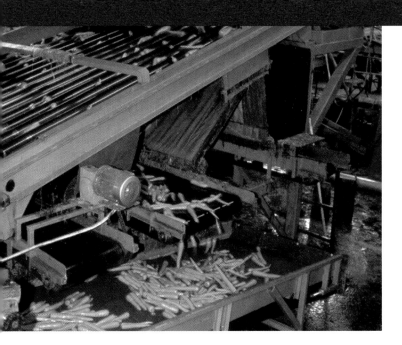

3 A Mechanical Soil and Gravel Separator

Problem Situation

Earth that is dug up often contains a mixture of many different particle sizes, from tiny clay particles to large pieces of gravel. However, gardeners and landscapers need these substances separated so that they are usable. For example, the gravel is useful for driveways or walkways; gardeners need clay to improve sandy soil; and so on.

Design Brief

- Design and build a separating device that efficiently separates the particles in stony soil into three different sizes.

Design Criteria

- The separating device must be capable of separating at least 1 kg of soil.
- The separator must collect each of the three different-sized particles in separate compartments.
- The separator must work without being touched directly by a human operator.

 When preparing to build or test a design, have your plan approved by your teacher before you begin.

Unit 1 Summary

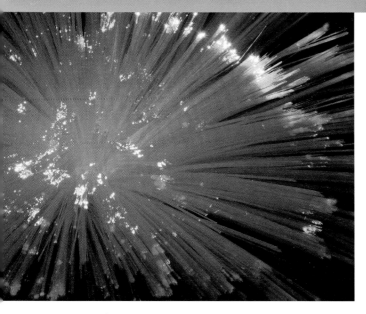

Reflecting

- Reflect on the ideas and questions presented in the Unit Overview and in the Getting Started. How can you connect what you have done and learned in this unit with those ideas and questions? (To review, check the sections indicated in this Summary.)
- Revise your answers to the Reflecting questions in ❶, ❷, ❸ and the questions you created in the Getting Started. How has your thinking changed?
- What new questions do you have? How will you answer them?

Understanding Concepts

- distinguish between pure substances, mechanical mixtures, and solutions using the particle theory 1.1, 1.2

- use the particle theory to explain how substances dissolve, based on attractions between the particles of solute and solvent 1.2, 1.5

- describe the difference between saturated and unsaturated solutions, between dilute and concentrated solutions 1.8, 1.9

- identify factors that affect the rate at which a substance dissolves 1.4, 1.7, 1.14

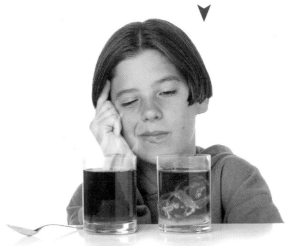

- identify solutes and solvents in various kinds of solutions 1.1, 1.11, 1.12

Applying Skills

- classify a sample of matter as a pure substance or a mixture; as a solution or a mechanical mixture 1.1, 1.2

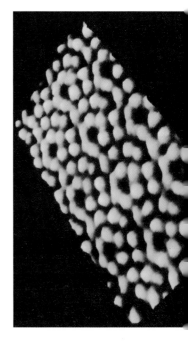

- conduct experiments to determine various factors that affect the rate at which substances dissolve 1.4, 1.7, 1.14

- determine the amount of solute required to form a saturated solution with a fixed amount of solvent at various temperatures 1.9

- investigate different methods of separating the components of mixtures 1.3, 1.10, 1.20

- evaluate the quality of water from different sources by performing simple tests 1.16, 1.17, 1.21

- identify different types of waste present in the community and the environmentally acceptable methods for their disposal 1.14, 1.15, 1.18

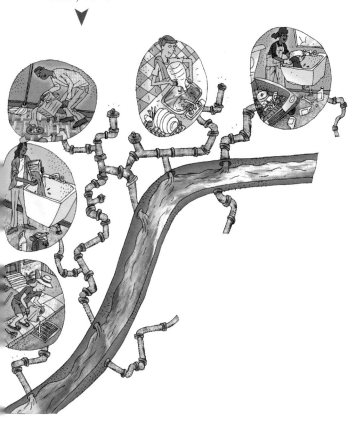

- understand and use the following terms:

alloy	plastic
ceramic	pure substance
concentrated solutions	raw material
dilute solutions	saturated solutions
glass	soft water
hard water	solubility
hazardous product	solute
heterogeneous mixture	solution
homogeneous mixture	solvent
matter	supersaturated
mechanical mixture	turbidity
mixture	unsaturated solutions
particle theory	WHMIS
pH scale	

Making Connections

- recognize that solutions in manufactured products can exist as solids, liquids, and gases 1.1, 1.11, 1.12

- distinguish between raw materials and manufactured products 1.12, 1.13

- identify a variety of manufactured products made from mixtures and explain their functions 1.6, 1.12, 1.13

- describe how raw materials are collected and processed to produce a variety of products 1.12, 1.13

- identify the sources and characteristics of pollutants that result from manufacturing and agricultural processes 1.15, 1.19

- describe the effects of some toxic solvents on the environment and regulations that ensure their safe use and disposal 1.18

- demonstrate the use of water as a solvent and as a chemical reactant 1,1, 1.4, 1.6, 1.10, 1.13, 1.14, 1.15, 1.17, 1.21

- evaluate how human use of natural resources has affected water systems 1.4, 1.17

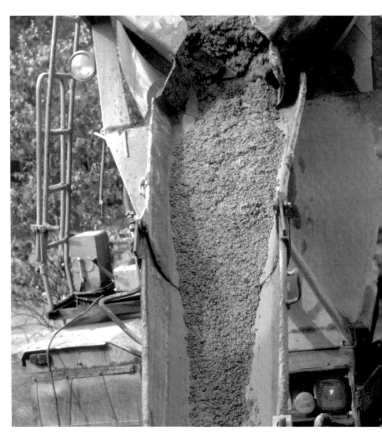

Unit 1 Review

Understanding Concepts

1. Copy the terms in Column A into your notebook. Match each term with the most correct description from Column B.

Column A	Column B
mechanical mixture	a solute that "disappears" in a solvent
solvent	mix together very well
solute	a tiny bit of solute in a large amount of solvent
concentration	contains more dissolved material than is required for saturation, at that temperature
dissolve	something in which a substance dissolves
insoluble	the mass of dissolved material in a specified amount of solvent
dilute	all spaces between solvent particles filled with solute
saturated	two or more pure substances in the same container
unsaturated	the substance that gets dissolved
soluble	mix together very well

2. State, with a reason, whether each of the following is a solution or a mechanical mixture:

   (a) hotdog relish

   (b) freshly squeezed grapefruit juice

   (c) soda water

   (d) apple juice

   (e) granola

   (f) vegetable soup

3. Decide whether each of the following is a solution or not. Give reasons for your choice.

   (a) a mixture of clay and water

   (b) a mixture of salt and water

   (c) tomato juice

4. Give examples of the following:
   (a) two pure substances
   (b) two solid solutions
   (c) two liquid solutions that do not contain water
   (d) a solution that is a gas

5. Is an alloy a pure substance or a mixture? Use the particle theory to explain your answer.

6. How do each of the following affect the solubility of a solid solute in water?

   (a) temperature

   (b) stirring

7. The Moon was once believed to have no water anywhere on its surface. If this were true, could there be solutions on the Moon? Explain.

8. Read the following statements. Rewrite those that are incorrect so that they become correct.

   (a) If a solution is saturated at 20°C, it will also be saturated at 25°C.

   (b) When some solvent evaporates, a solution becomes more saturated.

   (c) When a saturated solution is cooled, some crystals begin to appear in the solution. The solution is now unsaturated.

   (d) A solvent is a liquid that dissolves sugar.

   (e) A solute is always a solid.

   (f) Dissolving means mixing two things together.

   (g) Oil is insoluble.

9. Describe the information that you would obtain from each of the labels below

   (a)

   (b)

   (c)

10. Use the particle theory to explain

   (a) the difference between a pure substance and a mixture

   (b) the difference between a solution and a mechanical mixture

   (c) how a small amount of sugar dissolves in a container of water.

11. Identify a solute and the solvent in each of the following solutions:

   (a) salt water

   (b) air

   (c) brass

   (d) steel

12. What is the ideal pH for fresh water? Why? What is the effect on fresh water organisms if the water becomes too acidic? How are some bodies of water able to offset acidic precipitation? Explain your answers.

13. Why are each of the following added to drinking water?

   (a) chlorine

   (b) fluoride

14. What does the term "hazardous" mean when it is used to describe a substance? You dump a small amount of paint thinner down the drain before putting the can at the curb for recycling. Are you being environmentally responsible? State your reasons.

15. You add one teaspoon of lemon juice to a 400-mL cup of water. A friend adds four teaspoons of lemon juice to her 400-mL cup of water. Into whose cup would more sugar need to be added to make the drink sweet? Explain.

16. A perfume chemist determines that 5 g of Brand X perfume can dissolve in 50 g of water at room temperature. She also finds that 10 g of Brand Y perfume can dissolve in 100 g of water. She concludes that Brand Y perfume is more soluble in water than Brand X. Do you agree with her findings? Explain.

Applying Skills

17. Using a flashlight, how can you distinguish between a solution and a mechanical mixture ?

18. Prakesh makes the following entry in her notebook: "On Friday we were given a clear blue liquid in a shallow container. We placed it on the windowsill over the weekend. On Monday morning, there was no liquid left, but the dish had some solid blue stuff in it."

   (a) Was the blue liquid in the dish a heterogeneous mixture, a solution, or a pure substance? Design a procedure to verify your choice.

   (b) Write a hypothesis to account for what happened in the dish.

19. Use the solubility data for solid potassium nitrate in water at various temperatures from **Table 1**. Graph the data and answer the following questions.

Table 1

Temperature (°C)	0	10	20	30	40	50	60
Solubility of potassium nitrate (g solute/100g water)	14	21	31	45	60	85	110

   (a) How many grams of potassium nitrate will dissolve in 100 g of water at 30°C? At 35°C?

   (b) At what temperature will 40 g of potassium nitrate dissolve in 100 g of water to form a saturated solution?

   (c) At what temperature will 85 g of potassium nitrate dissolve in 100 g of water to form a saturated solution?

   (d) If 30 g of potassium nitrate are dissolved in 100 g of water at 18°C, is the solution saturated? Explain.

20. Use the data provided in **Table 1** in 1.8 to draw the solubility graphs for both sugar and salt. Use the graphs to answer the following questions.

   (a) How much sugar will dissolve to form a saturated solution in 100 g of water at 60°C? Salt?

   (b) If 20 g of salt is completely dissolved in 100 g of water at 50°C, what kind of solution will result?

21. Genna decides that, while she brushes her teeth, the tap should only be running while the toothbrush is being rinsed. She decides to investigate how much water is used if the tap is left running all the time she brushes. To her surprise, the extra water fills one 1.75-L bottle, along with half of another. If she brushes three times daily, how much water will Genna save in a year by turning off the tap?

22. A laboratory receives a bottle of red liquid for analysis. After it sits overnight, bits of red powder are found on the bottom of the container. When lab technicians shine a light into the container, the top of the beam appears pink, while the bottom appears red. Tiny particles are also observed in the beam of light. Does this bottle contain a solution? Explain.

23. Suggest a method to separate each of the following mixtures:

    (a) sand, salt, and bird seed

    (b) sugar, flour, and pennies

    (c) water and salad oil

    (d) iron powder, salt, and iron nails

24. Michael's results in a dissolving investigation are not consistent with the results of other students in the class. For solute 1, Michael half-filled a test tube with tap water, put in some solute, and then shook the test tube until his arm got tired. For solute 2, he put 5 mL of water into a beaker, added two crystals of solute 2, and stirred the contents once or twice with a stir stick.

    (a) What would you suggest to Michael to improve his experimental technique?

    (b) Effram and Michael argued over solute 3. Effram described it as "not very soluble." Michael insisted that it is "insoluble." How might you determine who is right?

25. Water is used to deliver fluoride to the citizens of a community because it is an excellent "carrier." What makes water such a good carrier?

Making Connections

26. Why does air, a solution, feel much more humid on a hot day than on a cool one, even if the relative humidity on both days is the same?

27. A good angel food cake does not appear to have any icing. Your grandmother tells you that she sprinkled some powdered sugar on the moist cake when it came out of the oven. What happened to it?

28. A student carefully removes the cap from a chilled bottle of pop. The open top is covered with a balloon that is secured with tape. When she shakes the bottle, the balloon fills with gas. This sequence is repeated with an identical bottle of pop at room temperature.

    (a) Which balloon will fill with the greatest amount of gas? Explain.

    (b) How is the solubility of carbon dioxide gas related to the temperature of the beverage?

29. Galvanized nails are now used for most outdoor applications. Investigate how a metal is galvanized and determine whether galvanized nails are, in fact, an alloy.

30. Gases that dissolve in water can make it look cloudy. Will hot water or cold water likely produce a cloudy ice cube? Explain.

31. Laura observes her friend Ingrid preparing to make a glass of lemon iced tea from a drink mix. Ingrid first fills a tall glass with ice cubes. She then adds a spoonful of drink mix and two sugar cube to the glass before adding cold tap water. A considerable amount of undissolved solid remains at the bottom of the glass.

    (a) Describe four suggestions that Laura could make to reduce the amount of undissolved solid.

    (b) Is Ingrid's first drink saturated, unsaturated, or supersaturated? Explain.

    (c) If Laura's suggestions are taken and there is no evidence of undissolved solid in the glass, how would you now describe the drink?

32. If pure gold is described as 24 karat, then 18-karat gold must consist of 18 parts gold and 6 parts other metals, such as copper.

(a) Name the solute in 18-karat gold.

(b) Name the solvent.

(c) Bill's girlfriend gives him a pure gold chain for his birthday. After a few weeks of wearing it, his skin becomes discoloured under the chain. What advice would you give Bill?

33. Rock candy is made by dissolving sugar in warm water to form a saturated solution and then is allowed to cool.

(a) What is rock candy?

(b) Explain how it is formed based on what you know about saturated solutions.

34. Imagine that you are an industrial chemist. Part of your job is to think of new and useful mixtures that your company can make. Using the following list of substances and their properties, name three mixtures that you would make, inventing a use for each one.

Substance	Useful Property
A	sticks to plastic
B	is bright blue
C	boils at 20ºC
D	smells like bananas
E	is elastic
F	glows in the dark
G	conducts electricity
H	bends without breaking
I	repels insects

35. The instructions on an aerosol can of oven cleaner advises the user to wear rubber gloves while using the product. The can also contains two WHMIS warning labels. Which two?

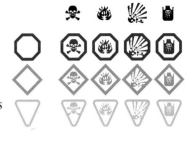

36. You decide to enter a competition to build a mountain bike that has no metal parts.

(a) What materials that you have learned about here would you use to replace the metal parts of your mountain bike? Explain the reasons for your choices.

(b) If you wanted to build a racing bike, would your choice of materials change? Explain.

37. Lake trout prefer oxygen-rich water. Where would you expect to find trout in mid-summer—at the bottom of the lake or near the surface?

38. A soup recipe calls for the addition of bouillon. A cook finds both bouillon powder and bouillon cubes in the spice cabinet. Which form of the substance will speed up the process of making the soup?

39. A large bottle of liquid laundry detergent states that it contains enough detergent to wash 100 loads of laundry. A different brand in a smaller bottle also states that it contains enough detergent to wash 100 loads of laundry. Both are true. Explain how this could be.

40. It is discovered that a newly developed chemical reduces the desire to eat. Politicians in a small municipality decide that it would be a good idea to add small amounts of this chemical to drinking water. They argue that dissolving the chemical in everyone's drinking water would result in a lowered demand on countries to produce food and would help overweight people lose weight. State your position on this issue. Give some reasons to support your position.

Glossary

A

alloy: a homogeneous mixture of two or more metals or metals and other substances in a solid solution

C

ceramic: a material manufactured by heating minerals and rocks; ceramics include pottery, bricks, cement, and glass

concentrated solution: a solution that contains a high amount of solute

D

diversity: a measure of the number of different types of organisms in an area

G

glass: a ceramic product made by mixing small amounts of limestone and potash with silica at high temperatures; a solution that is a supercooled liquid

H

hard water: water that contains certain dissolved substances, such as magnesium, calcium, or sulfur, which prevent soap from forming a lather

hazardous product: a substance that requires special handling and storage because it is dangerous to human health or to the environment

heterogeneous mixture: an uneven mixture that contains two or more substances; samples of heterogeneous mixture may have different properties

homogeneous mixture: a mixture that is the same throughout; all samples taken from a homogeneous mixture (a solution) will have the same properties

M

matter: anything that takes up space and has mass

mechanical mixture: a heterogeneous mixture; in a mechanical mixture at least two substances are visible

mixture: any substance that contains at least two pure substances

P

particle theory: a theory used to explain matter and heat transfer. It suggests that all matter is made up of tiny particles too small to be seen. These particles are constantly in motion because they have energy. The more energy they have, the faster they move.

pH scale: a gauge, ranging from 0 (strongly acidic) to 14 (strongly alkaline), used to express the acidity or alkalinity of a solution

plastic: a modern material manufactured in a multistep process, beginning with oil and gas

pure substance: any solid, liquid, or gas that contains only one kind of particle throughout.

R

raw material: unprocessed material of any kind

S

saturated solution: a solution that contains the maximum amount of solute that the solvent can dissolve at the given temperature

soft water: water that contains very small amounts of dissolved minerals; easily forms a lather when mixed with soap

solubility: the maximum amount of a particular solute that can be dissolved in a particular solvent at a given temperature

solute: a substance that is dissolved in a solvent to form a solution

solution: a homogeneous mixture made of a solvent and one or more solutes; in a solution, only one substance is visible; a solution can be solid, liquid, or gas

solvent: a substance that dissolves a solute to form a solution

supersaturated solution: a solution that contains more of the solute than would be found in a saturated solution

T

turbidity: a measure of the amount of suspended solids in water, calculated using special meters

U

unsaturated solution: a solution in which more solute can be dissolved at the given temperature

W

WHMIS: (Workplace Hazardous Materials Information System) symbols found on hazardous products that identify the type of danger associated with the product and provide information on safe handling

Index